Case Studies in Movement Disorders

Case Studies in Movement Disorders

Common and Uncommon Presentations

Edited by

Roberto Erro
Center for Neurodegenerative Diseases (CEMAND), Department of Medicine and Surgery, Neuroscience Section, University of Salerno, Italy
Sobell Department of Movement Disorders and Motor Neuroscience, Institute of Neurology, UCL, London, UK

Maria Stamelou
University of Athens Medical School, 2nd Department of Neurology, Hospital Attikon, Athens, Greece
Movement Disorders Department, HYGEIA Hospital, Athens, Greece
Department of Neurology, Philipps University, Marburg, Germany

Kailash P. Bhatia
Sobell Department of Movement Disorders and Motor Neuroscience, Institute of Neurology, UCL, London, UK

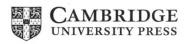

CAMBRIDGE
UNIVERSITY PRESS

CAMBRIDGE
UNIVERSITY PRESS

University Printing House, Cambridge CB2 8BS, United Kingdom
One Liberty Plaza, 20th Floor, New York, NY 10006, USA
477 Williamstown Road, Port Melbourne, VIC 3207, Australia
4843/24, 2nd Floor, Ansari Road, Daryaganj, Delhi – 110002, India
79 Anson Road, #06-04/06, Singapore 079906

Cambridge University Press is part of the University of Cambridge.

It furthers the University's mission by disseminating knowledge in the pursuit of
education, learning, and research at the highest international levels of excellence.

www.cambridge.org
Information on this title: www.cambridge.org/9781107472426
DOI: 10.1017/9781316145050

© Cambridge University Press 2017

First published 2017

Printed in the United Kingdom by TJ International Ltd. Padstow Cornwall

A catalogue record for this publication is available from the British Library.

Library of Congress Cataloging-in-Publication Data
Names: Bhatia, Kailash, editor. | Erro, Roberto, editor. | Stamelou, Maria, editor.
Title: Case studies in movement disorders: common and uncommon presentations / edited by Kailash Bhatia, Sobell Department of
Movement Disorders and Motor Neuroscience, UCL Institute of Neurology, London, UK, Roberto Erro, Center for Neurodegenerative
Diseases (CEMAND), Department of Medicine and Surgery, Neuroscience Section, University of Salerno, Italy, Sobell Department of
Movement Disorders and Motor Neuroscience, UCL Institute of Neurology, London, UK, Maria Stamelou, University of Athens Medical
School, 2nd Department of Neurology, Hospital Attikon, Athens, Greece, Department of Neurology, Philipps University, Marburg, Germany.
Description: Cambridge, United Kingdom; New York, NY: Cambridge University Press, 2017. |
Includes bibliographical references and index.
Identifiers: LCCN 2017000344 | ISBN 9781107472426 (paperback)
Subjects: LCSH: Movement disorders. | Movement disorders – Case studies. | BISAC: MEDICAL / Neurology.
Classification: LCC RC376.5.C375 2017 | DDC 616.8/3–dc23
LC record available at https://lccn.loc.gov/2017000344

ISBN 978-1-107-47242-6 Paperback

....

Every effort has been made in preparing this book to provide accurate and up-to-date information that
is in accord with accepted standards and practice at the time of publication. Although case histories are
drawn from actual cases, every effort has been made to disguise the identities of the individuals
involved. Nevertheless, the authors, editors, and publishers can make no warranties that the
information contained herein is totally free from error, not least because clinical standards are
constantly changing through research and regulation. The authors, editors, and publishers
therefore disclaim all liability for direct or consequential damages resulting from the use of
material contained in this book. Readers are strongly advised to pay careful attention to
information provided by the manufacturer of any drugs or equipment that they plan to use.

Contents

The colour plates appear between pages 100 and 101.

Video Captions

The following is a list of captions relating to videos cited in individual cases. Please see the URL at the end of this list for a link to the video content.

1.1 The video sequence shows a 70-year-old patient with left-sided resting tremor. There is also a mild left-sided postural and action tremor. His finger and foot tapping are bradykinetic on his left side with some interruptions of the motor sequences. On his right side, his movements are also irregular with occasional interruptions, but there is no clear fatiguing. His shoulder shrug is reduced on his left. On walking, his arm swing is decreased on his left with rest tremor appearing, while the pattern of his gait is quite normal.   2

3.1 Abnormal posturing of the right foot, which is turned inwards. The dystonic posturing improves when the patient walks backwards or with his knees flexed.   6

4.1 Left-sided rest tremor of the upper and lower limb. Bradykinesia on finger tapping is shown on the left. Gait is reasonably long stepped, but arm swing is reduced.   8

5.1 Segment 1: gait showing broad base with instability and backwards fall after turning 180 degrees; Segment 2: postural instability; Segment 3: two years later there is marked worsening of gait; Segment 4: restriction of downwards gaze; Segment 5: bradykinesia; Segment 6: speech abnormalities.   11

6.1 Finger-tapping manoeuvre showing absence of decrement and bradykinesia.   14

7.1 Segment 1: delayed ocular saccades with associated head thrusts; Segment 2: apraxic pattern of gait; Segment 3: oro-buccal and limb apraxia, action myoclonus and magnetism of the left arm   17

8.1 Segment 1: broken pursuit eye movements with associated gaze-evoked nystagmus and dysmetric saccades; Segment 2: bilateral bradykinesia; Segment 3: limb ataxia with dysmetria and dysdiadochokinesia.   19

9.1 Speech stuttering and freezing of gait, mainly on turning.   23

10.1 There is frontalis overcativity and she has a staring expression. Ocular movements are very restricted upwards, but only partially correctable with the eye-doll manoeuvre. There is no clear appendicular bradykinesia.   25

11.1 This patient has reduced blink rate and a retrocollis. On finger tapping there is bradykinesia (left>right). He walks with a stooped posture and short steps. Arm swing is reduced and arms are held in a flexed position.   28

12.1 There is an irregular rest tremor of the right hand, along with an asymmetric bilateral tremor (right>left) and dystonic posturing of the hands on posture. Moreover, there is a mild bradykinesia of the right hand. There is some difficulty with copying gestures particularly with her left hand.   30

13.1 There is frontalis overactivity and the patient has a staring expression. Ocular pursuits are restricted on the vertical plane. Saccades are slow and hypometric on the vertical plane as compared to the horizontal one. There is bradykinesia, especially on the left and frontal release signs. Gait is impossible with support, also owing to severe imbalance.   32

14.1 This patient is wheelchair bound. She has hypomimia and a laterocollis to the right. There is a tremor in her right arm on posture and there is marked hypokinesia.   34

16.1 This patient has a generalized dystonia affecting her trunk and lower limbs, with evident tremor. Her gait is dystonic and affected by the trunk involvement.   41

17.1 There is a generalized dystonia with a superimposed jerky tremor, most evident in her upper limbs and neck. Her gait is dystonic and affected by superimposed jerks of her trunk. 43

18.1 There is generalized dystonia with prominent oromandibular involvement and tongue enlargement. Dystonia is also seen in her arms, trunk and lower limbs, particularly the left one. 45

19.1 There is generalized dystonia, mainly involving his cervical region and trunk. He also has facial grimacing and platysma overactivity. There are dystonic movements of his head and arms on posture, with an additional jerking component. The abnormal posturing of his right arm can be best appreciated on writing. 47

20.1 This patient has a left foot dystonia, which is turned inwards and affects his walking. Note the callosity on the outer margin of the foot. There is mild dystonia in his upper limbs. 49

21.1 This patient has spontaneous myoclonic jerks in her face and both upper and lower limbs. There is a clear dysarthria, and dystonia is most evident in her neck and upper limbs. She is slow bilaterally on finger tapping. Unaided walking is impossible: her gait is impaired due to the presence of dystonic features in the lower limbs and truncal hypothonia. 51

22.1 This patient is in a wheelchair and is not able to stand and walk. He has macrocephaly and his speech is grossly dysarthric, with dystonia being the main component. He has generalized dystonia, which has affected the cranial region and the tongue. A fixed contracture of his left hand is seen and he could not use it at all; there is also evidence of mild weakness. 54

22.2 This patient with Glutaric Aciduria type 1 has a mild phenotype with hemi-dystonia that has affected the right side of his body and additional pyramidal signs in his right leg. 54

23.1 Prominent jaw-opening dystonia is shown. There is additional (mild) dystonic posturing in the upper limbs, where a postural tremor also occurs. Ocular movements on the vertical plane are restricted. Gait reflects a combination of dystonic and spastic features. 57

24.1 This patient has oromandibular dyskinesia with motor impersistence when asked to protrude her tongue out of her mouth. There is a bilateral postural tremor of her arms with additional chorea and dystonic posturing. She has freezing of gait, mainly on turning, and postural reflexes loss. 60

25.1 This patient has generalized dystonia with prominent oromandibular involvement and tongue protrusion. The video also shows one episode of neck turning and eye version, suggestive of an oculogyric crisis. Both feet are everted, and an extensor plantar response of the left foot is shown. He has a patch of scopolamine for excessive drooling. 62

27.1 There is generalized dystonia with prominent oromandubular involvement and facial grimacing. She is aphonic and cannot protrude her tongue. There is mild ataxia on finger–nose test and a terminal tremor bilaterally. She has difficulties in performing repetitive movements, particularly with her right hand. Unaided walking is impossible. Bilateral extensor plantar reflex is shown. 66

28.1 There is a severe retrocollis as well as a mild extensor trunk dystonia. This patient has to hold his head tight to not lose his balance when walking. 68

30.1 Patient is being filmed while alone in room. Video demonstrates a repertoire of multiple simple and complex motor and phonic tics. 72

31.1 Patient gives brief description of his medical history. Video demonstrates multiple simple and complex motor tics, as well as prominent simple phonic tics and generalized chorea. He also appears restless (he had not been treated with neuroleptics). Hyperkinetic movements are only partially suppressible for a very brief period of time (<5 seconds). There is no bradykinesia or upper limb ataxia. Gait appears stiff with clear dystonic posturing of the right leg. 74

32.1 A: classic, short lasting (<10 seconds in this segment) paroxysmal kinesigenic dyskinesia attack with generalized dystonic choreic-ballistic movements. B: hyperactive patient is being filmed while alone in room. Video demonstrates multiple simple and complex motor tics, as well as simple phonic tics. 77

33.1 Brief, sudden, repetitive, and phenomenologically invariable movements consisting of neck flexion, loud vocalizations, and arm flinging, when fully conscious. In one of these episodes the patient describes his awareness of a building pressure/pain in his head prior to the episode.   79

34.1 This patient has difficulties initiating saccades and has to blink to defixate. Moreover, there are choreic movements affecting his face and upper limbs.   82

35.1 There is generalized chorea with truncal movements. He has prominent orobulbar involvement with marked dysarthria with bruxism and tongue biting. His gait is very unstable and lurching.   84

36.1 There is mild chorea in her arms that is also interfering with repetitive finger movements. There is motor impersistence on tongue protrusion. Finger–nose testing shows very mild upper limb ataxia. She has a wide-based gait, and tandem gait is almost impossible.   86

37.1 Abnormal eye movements with poor gaze initiation, impaired pursuit, saccadic hypometria with head thrusts, and reduced vertical up-gaze. There is generalized chorea with myoclonic movements of the head and neck. Gait is slightly broad based, with reduced arm swing and with both arms tending to hold slightly dystonic postures. During gait, facial and oro-buccal choreic movements can be seen.   88

38.1 Besides the generalized dystonia, there are generalized choreiform movements involving his face, arms, legs, and toes that are not predictable or patterned.   90

39.1 This patient has moderate choreic dyskinesias mainly affecting his lower limbs and additional abnormal posturing of his neck and trunk. His gait is mildly unsteady and there is reduced arm swing. Postural reflexes are preserved.   92

40.1 There is motor impersistence on tongue protrusion. Generalized choreic movements are seen mainly in the upper limbs but also in the lower ones and toes. There is also mild dystonic posturing of the fingers bilaterally.   94

41.1 There is generalized chorea with superimposed dystonic posturing, with clear torticollis to the left. Gait is unsteady with both choreiform and dystonic features.   96

42.1 There is no tremor at rest. A fine symmetrical tremor of his arms can be seen on posture, with no evidence of dystonia. The tremor is more evident on action (finger–nose test, writing, pouring water from one glass to another).   98

43.1 She is hypomimic. There is a rest tremor of her right hand. A bilateral postural tremor of her arms is shown, with no re-emergence. There is no bradykinesia.   100

44.1 There is a bilateral, symmetric postural fine tremor of the upper limbs with no dystonic posturing, while no tremor is seen at rest and on action.   102

45.1 This patient has a postural tremor (left>right) when his arms are outstretched in front of him. However, his tremor changes pattern and increases in amplitude on his right arm with elbow flexed (wing position). There is also a bilateral action tremor as well as head titubation.   104

46.1 Irregular fast tremor of the right hand at rest and on posture is shown.   106

48.1 Palatal tremor which completely stops when the patient is asked to tap with her fingers.   110

49.1 This patient has a mild torticollis and laterocollis with associated head tremor at about 4 Hz. Irregular jaw and lip tremor during neck extension is seen. She has adductor-type dystonic voice tremor and an irregular, jerky tongue tremor as well as facial (eyebrow/perioral) tremor. Jerky dystonic arm tremor and dystonic hand posturing (right>left) is seen. In addition, she has bilateral intention tremor, decomposition of movement on finger–nose test, and a megalographic dysgraphia.   112

50.1 A bilateral rest, postural, and action tremor with low frequency and high amplitude is seen.   114

51.1 There is a tremor of his right arm only on writing, while no tremor can be seen at rest, on posture, or on action.   116

52.1 Generalized myoclonus is shown, with clear retrocollic 'shock-like' as well as less brusque proximal limb jerks. The jerks are not stimulus sensitive. He also has a slight torticollis to the right.   118

54.1 The video shows the patient at age 55. She is confined to the wheelchair. There are generalized myoclonic jerks (affecting face, neck, arms, and to a lesser degree legs), which become much more pronounced on action or even with visual stimuli. For example, during smooth pursuit eye movements, the jerks affecting her neck become quite violent. There is mild end-gaze nystagmus. When holding her arms outstretched, positive and negative myoclonus impedes her holding the arms still and interferes with testing for dysmetria. Myoclonus can be elicited by light touch. Other features comprise abolished deep tendon reflexes and scoliosis.   122

55.1 Stimulus-sensitive myoclonus is shown both in upper and lower limbs. There is also action myoclonus when the patient attempts to put his socks on and gait ataxia without limb ataxia.   124

56.1 The video shows bradykinesia on finger tapping with the right hand. Stimulus-sensitive myoclonus of the right limbs as well as apraxia of the right hand are shown.   126

58.1 This patient has myoclonic twitches on the right side of the face, mainly in the lower part, when speaking. His voice is also affected, and he tends to stutter when his facial twitches occur. He has a fine jerky tremor of his both arms on posture. Myoclonic jerks are evident in his lower limbs when he is asked to stand on one leg.   130

59.1 There is a myoclonic tremor on posture of his arms and legs. Furthermore, his tongue shakes when protruded.   132

60.1 This patient has repetitive jerks originating from the trunk and propagating to his lower limbs.   134

62.1 She has a scanning speech and broken smooth pursuit. There is bradykinesia on finger tapping bilaterally. Limb ataxia is shown on finger–nose test. Her gait is short-stepped, but also wide based.   138

63.1 A bilateral, though asymmetric, irregular tremor is seen at rest, on posture and action. Moreover, there is general hypokinesia, although it is difficult to judge whether there is decrement on finger tapping, also because tremor frequency tends to take over during finger tapping. Gait is unstable and reflects a combination of parkinsonian and ataxic features.   140

64.1 There is an almost complete ophthalmoplegia on both horizontal and vertical plane. Gait is short-stepped and an episode of freezing occurs.   142

65.1 There is dystonia, most prominent in her cervical region, with a sensory trick. Mild posturing and dystonic movements are seen in her upper limbs. There is no evidence of limb or gait ataxia. On the posterior pharyngeal wall, a telangiectasia can be seen.   144

65.2 Smooth pursuits are broken and there is gaze-evoked nystagmus as well as leashes of telangiectasia in the bulbar conjunctiva in both eyes. There is also mild ataxia and dysdiadochokinesia in the upper limbs.   144

66.1 There is limb ataxia more pronounced on the right, as well as a cerebellar tremor more on the right with slow frequency and high amplitude.   146

67.1 A: This patient has truncal ataxia as well as upper limb dysmetria (left>right) and dysdiadochokinesis. There is leg spasticity with prominent involvement of the hip adductors. Spastic-ataxic gait with prominent truncal ataxia is shown. B: Same patient 6 months later after having been treated with botulinum toxin injections into both long adductor muscles.   148

To access video content, please visit www.cambridge.org/9781107472426.

Contributors

Elena Antelmi
Sobell Department of Movement Disorders and
Motor Neuroscience, Institute of Neurology, UCL,
London, UK

Department of Biomedical and Neuromotor Sciences,
Alma Mater Studiorum, University of Bologna,
Bologna, Italy

IRCSS, Institute of Neurological Sciences,
Bologna, Italy

Bettina Balint
Sobell Department of Movement Disorders and
Motor Neuroscience, Institute of Neurology, UCL,
London, UK

Department of Neurology, University Hospital
Heidelberg, Heidelberg, Germany

Pedro Barbosa
Queen Square Brain Bank for Neurological Disorders,
Institute of Neurology, UCL, London, UK

Reta Lila Weston Institute of Neurological Studies,
Institute of Neurology, UCL, London, UK

Paolo Barone
Center for Neurodegenerative Diseases (CEMAND),
Department of Medicine and Surgery, Neuroscience
Section, University of Salerno, Italy

Amit Batla
Sobell Department of Movement Disorders and
Motor Neuroscience, UCL Institute of Neurology,
London, UK

Kailash P. Bhatia
Sobell Department of Movement Disorders and
Motor Neuroscience, Institute of Neurology, UCL,
London, UK

Florian Brugger
Klinik für Neurologie, Kantonsspital St. Gallen,
Switzerland

Sobell Department of Movement Disorders and
Motor Neuroscience, Institute of Neurology, UCL,
London, UK

Carla Cordivari
National Hospital for Neurology and Neurosurgery,
London, UK

George Dervenoulas
University of Athens Medical School, 2nd Department
of Neurology, Hospital Attikon, Athens, Greece

Roberto Erro
Center for Neurodegenerative Diseases (CEMAND),
Department of Medicine and Surgery, Neuroscience
Section, University of Salerno, Italy

Sobell Department of Movement Disorders and
Motor Neuroscience, Institute of Neurology, UCL,
London, UK

Christos Ganos
Sobell Department of Motor Neuroscience and
Movement Disorders, Institute of Neurology, UCL,
London, UK

Department of Neurology, University Medical Center
Hamburg-Eppendorf (UKE), Hamburg, Germany

Davina J. Hensman Moss
Department of Neurodegenerative Disease, Institute
of Neurology, UCL, London, UK

Stephanie T. Hirschbichler
Sobell Department of Movement Disorders and
Motor Neuroscience, Institute of Neurology, UCL,
London, UK

Janice Holton

Queen Square Brain Bank for Neurological Disorders, Institute of Neurology, UCL, London, UK

Department of Molecular Neuroscience & Neurogenetics Laboratory, Institute of Neurology, UCL, London, UK

Henry Houlden

Department of Molecular Neuroscience & Neurogenetics Laboratory, Institute of Neurology, UCL, London, UK

Zane Jaunmuktane

Division of Neuropathology & Department of Neurodegenerative Disease, Institute of Neurology, UCL, London, UK

Helen Ling

Queen Square Brain Bank for Neurological Disorders, Institute of Neurology, UCL, London, UK

Reta Lila Weston Institute of Neurological Studies, Institute of Neurology, UCL, London, UK

David S. Lynch

Department of Molecular Neuroscience, Institute of Neurology, UCL, London, UK

Eduardo de Pablo-Fernandez

Queen Square Brain Bank for Neurological Disorders, Institute of Neurology, UCL, London, UK

Reta Lila Weston Institute of Neurological Studies, Institute of Neurology, UCL, London, UK

Tamas Revesz

Queen Square Brain Bank for Neurological Disorders, Institute of Neurology, UCL, London, UK

Maria Stamelou

University of Athens Medical School, 2nd Department of Neurology, Hospital Attikon, Athens, Greece

Movement Disorders Department., HYGEIA Hospital, Athens, Greece

Department of Neurology, Philipps University, Marburg, Germany

Leonidas Stefanis

University of Athens Medical School, 2nd Department of Neurology, Hospital Attikon, Athens, Greece

Biomedical Research Foundation of the Academy of Athens, Athens, Greece

Sarah J. Tabrizi

Department of Neurodegenerative Disease, Institute of Neurology, UCL, London, UK

Thomas Warner

Queen Square Brain Bank for Neurological Disorders, Institute of Neurology, UCL, London, UK

Reta Lila Weston Institute of Neurological Studies, Institute of Neurology, UCL, London, UK

Preface

Most books on movement disorders have a traditional approach with chapters on various topics. However, movement disorders is one area of neurology that is most dependent on the examination and clinical reasoning in a given case. Therefore, we felt it could be valuable to achieve learning through sharing our experience in a great number of movement disorders cases, taking the reader through the process of diagnosis and investigation based on clinical features. For this purpose, the cases in this book were selected to illustrate common and uncommon presentations of both more frequent and rare movement disorders. Through the chapters we have tried to project a way of thinking to arrive at the diagnosis using appropriate investigations, as we do in our clinical practice. General and special remarks will guide the reader through the differential diagnosis of each individual case and further provide general information on each individual disorder covered in that chapter.

We feel that *Case Studies in Movement Disorders* will be of immense benefit not only to students, residents and all who are new to the field, but also to established neurologists and those with experience in movement disorders alike.

We would like to thank our patients for their unwavering commitment to research and teaching activities. We also express our gratitude to all the contributors who shared with us their invaluable experience in this book.

Previously Published Cases

Case 9 Stamelou M, Kojovic M, Edwards MJ, Bhatia KP. Ability to cycle despite severe freezing of gait in atypical parkinsonism in Fahr's syndrome. *Mov Disord*. 2011;26:2141–2

Case 12 Hirschbichler ST, Erro R, Batla A, Bhatia KP. Classic PD-like rest tremor associated with the tau p.R406W mutation. *Parkinsonism Relat Disord*. 2015;21:1002–4

Case 13 Erro R, Lees AJ, Moccia M et al. Progressive parkinsonism, balance difficulties, and supranuclear gaze palsy. *JAMA Neurol*. 2014;71(1):104–7

Case 23 Kojovic M, Kuoppamäki M, Quinn N, Bhatia KP. 'Progressive delayed-onset postanoxic dystonia' diagnosed with PANK2 mutations 26 years after onset – an update. *Mov Disord*. 2010;25:2889–91

Case 27 Erro R, Hersheson J, Ganos C et al. H-ABC syndrome and DYT4: variable expressivity or pleiotropy of TUBB4 mutations? *Mov Disord*. 2015;30:828–33

Case 32 Ganos C, Mencacci N, Gardiner A et al. Paroxysmal kinesigenic dyskinesia may be misdiagnosed in co-occurring Gilles de la Tourette syndrome. *Mov Disord Clin Pract* 2014;1:84–6.

Case 35 Schneider SA, Lang AE, Moro E, Bader B, Danek A, Bhatia KP. Characteristic head drops and axial extension in advanced chorea-acanthocytosis. *Mov Disord*. 2010;25:1487–91

Case 36 Schneider SA, van de Warrenburg BP, Hughes TD et al. Phenotypic homogeneity of the Huntington disease-like presentation in a SCA17 family. *Neurology* 2006;67:1701–3.

Case 37 Hensman Moss DJ, Poulter M, Beck J et al. C9orf72 expansions are the most common genetic cause of Huntington disease phenocopies. *Neurology*. 2014;82:292–9.

Case 38 Antelmi E, Erro R, Pisani A, Mencacci N, Bhatia KP. Persistent chorea in DYT6, due to anticholinergic therapy. *Parkinsonism Relat Disord*. 2015;21:1282–3.

Case 41 Mencacci NE, Erro R, Wiethoff S et al. ADCY5 mutations are another cause of benign hereditary chorea. *Neurology* 2015;85:80–8.

Case 49 Ganos C, Saifee TA, Kassavetis P et al. Dystonic tremor and spasmodic dysphonia in spinocerebellar ataxia type 12. *Mov Disord Clin Pract* 2014;1:79–81.

Case 51 Erro R, Ciocca M, Hirschbichler ST, Rothwell JC, Bhatia KP. Primary writing tremor is a dystonic trait: evidence from an instructive family. *J Neurol Sci*. 2015;356:210–1.

Case 54 Praschberger R, Balint B, Mencacci NE et al. Expanding the phenotype and genetic defects associated with the GOSR2 gene. *Mov Disord Clin Pract* 2015;2:271–3

Case 64 Batla A, Erro R, Ganos C, Stamelou M, Bhatia KP. Levodopa-responsive Parkinsonism with prominent freezing and abnormal dopamine transporter scan associated with SANDO syndrome. *Mov Disord Clin Pract* 2015;3:304–7.

Case 65 Carrillo F, Schneider SA, Taylor AM et al. Prominent oromandibular dystonia and pharyngeal telangiectasia in atypical ataxia telangiectasia. *Cerebellum* 2009;8:22–7.

Abbreviations

AD	Alzheimer Disease	FDG-PET	Fludeoxyglucose-PET
ADHD	Attention Deficit/Hyperactivity Disorder	FHM	Familial Hemiplegic Migraine
A&E	Accidents & Emergencies	FLAIR	Fluid Attenuation Inversion Recovery
AFP	Alpha-Fetoprotein	FMD	Functional Movement Disorders
ASD	Autism Spectrum Disorder	FOG	Freezing of Gait
AT	Ataxia Telangiectasia	FTD	Frontotemporal Dementia
ATM	Ataxia Telangiectasia Mutated	FTDP-17	Frontotemporal Dementia Linked to Chromosome 17
BHC	Benign Hereditary Chorea		
BP	Bereitschaftspotential	FTLD	Frontotemporal Lobar Degeneration
BSE	Bovine Spongiform Encephalopathy	FXTAS	Fragile X Tremor-Ataxia Syndrome
CAG	Cytosine-Adenine-Guanine	GABA	Gamma-Aminobutyric Acid
CBD	Corticobasal Degeneration	GID	Graft-Induced Dyskinesias
CBS	Corticobasal Syndrome	GTCS	Generalized Tonic-Clonic Seizures
CADASIL	Ccerebral Autosomal Dominant Arteriopathy with Sub-cortical Infarcts and Leukoencephalopathy	GTS	Gilles de la Tourette Syndrome
		H-ABC	Hypomyelination with Atrophy of Basal Ganglia and Cerebellum
CANVAS	Cerebellar Ataxia with Neuropathy and Bilateral Vestibular Areflexia	HD	Huntington's Disease
		HDLS	Hereditary Diffuse Leukoencephalopathy with Axonal Spheroids
CEA	Carcinoembryonic Antigen		
CGG	Cytosine-Guanine-Guanine	HPRT	Hypoxanthine-Guanine Phosphoribosyltransferase
ChAc	Chorea-Acanthocytosis		
CIDP	Chronic Inflammatory Demyelinating Polyneuropathy	HSP	Hereditary Spastic Paraplegias
		ILOCA	Idiopathic Late Onset Cerebellar Ataxia
CJD	Creutzfeldt-Jakob Disease	JME	Juvenile Myoclonic Epilepsy
CK	Creatine-Kinase	LID	Levodopa-Induced Dyskinesias
CNS	Central Nervous System	MERRF	Myoclonic Epilepsy with Ragged Red Fibers
CP	Cerebral Palsy		
CSF	Cerebrospinal Fluid	MMSE	Mini-Mental State Examination
DaT-Scan	Dopamine Transporter SPECT Scan	MND	Motor Neuron Disease
DBS	Deep Brain Stimulation	MRI	Magnetic Resonance Imaging
DRD	Dopa-Responsive Dystonia	MS	Multiple Sclerosis
DRPLA	Dentatorubropallidolusyan Atrophy	MSA	Multiple System Atrophy
DWI	Diffusion Weighted Imaging	MSA-C	Multiple System Atrophy Cerebellar Variant
EA	Episodic Ataxia		
EEG	Electroencephalography	MSA-P	Multiple System Atrophy Parkinsonian Variant
EMG	Electromyography		
ET	Essential Tremor	mtDNA	Mitochondrial DNA
FCMTE	Familial Cortical Myoclonic Tremor with Epilepsy	NBIA	Neurodegeneration with Brain Iron Accumulation
FDFM	Familial Dyskinesia and Facial Myokymia	NMDA	N-methyl-D-aspartate

NMS	Nonmotor Symptoms	PSP-P	Progressive Supranuclear Palsy-Parkinsonism
NPC	Niemann-Pick Disease Type C	PSP-RS	Progressive Supranuclear Palsy-Richardson Syndrome
NPH	Normal Pressure Hydrocephalus		
OCB	Obsessive-Compulsive Behaviours	PT	Palatal Tremor
OCD	Obsessive-Compulsive Disorder	PWT	Primary Writing Tremor
OPC	Olivopontocerebellar	RBD	REM Sleep Behaviour Disorder
OT	Orthostatic Tremor	SANDO	Sensory Ataxic Neuropathy with Dysarthria and Ophthalmoparesis
PAPT	Progressive Ataxia and Palatal Tremor		
PCR	Polymerase Chain Reaction	SCA	Spinocerebellar Ataxia
PD	Parkinson's Disease	SNCA	Alpha-Synuclein gene
PED	Paroxysmal Exercise-Induced Dystonia	SND	Striatonigral Degeneration
PEO	Progressive External Ophthalmoplegia	SSEP	Somatosensory Evoked Potentials
PET	Positron Emission Tomography	SSM	Segmental Spinal Myoclonus
PFBC	Primary Familial Brain Calcification	SWEDD	Scans without Evidence of Dopaminergic Deficit
PKAN	Pantothenate Kinase–Associated Neurodegeneration		
		SWI	Susceptibility Weighted Imaging
PKD	Paroxysmal Kinesigenic Dyskinesia	TD	Tardive Dyskinesias
PLAN	PLA2G6-Associated Neurodegeneration	TH	Tyrosine Hydroxylase
PMA	Progressive Myoclonic Ataxia	ULD	Unverricht-Lundborg Disease
PME	Progressive Myoclonic Epilepsy	VDRL	Venereal Disease Research Laboratory
PSM	Propriospinal Myoclonus	WD	Wilson's Disease
PSP	Progressive Supranuclear Palsy		

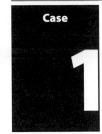

Case

1

Parkinson's Disease

Florian Brugger and Kailash P. Bhatia

Clinical History

A 70-year-old British man without family history for any neurological disorder was referred due to a tremor of his left hand. Initially, the tremor presented only when holding items, but then progressed over the subsequent years and also became more apparent during rest. Furthermore, he noticed that he had become slower in his day-to-day activities. There were some indications of having vivid dreams and acting out his dreams. He reported normal autonomic functions, and his memory was well preserved.

Examination

A left-sided resting tremor of about 4–5 Hz with a pill-rolling aspect was the most prominent clinical feature on examination (Video 1.1). Upon lifting his arms, his tremor briefly stopped, but then re-emerged thereafter. There was also a mild postural tremor on the left-hand side. His finger and foot tapping were slightly bradykinetic on the left-hand side with a mild decrease of amplitude and speed. There was mild cog-wheeling rigidity in his left arm. He had mildly reduced facial expression. His saccades were broken and slightly hypometric, but they were normal in speed, range and directory. His posture was slightly stooped. While walking, a reduced arm swing on the left side was the only abnormal feature. His clinical examination was otherwise unremarkable.

General Remarks

The asymmetric/unilateral hand tremor is the dominating clinical feature in this patient. In the first instance, this leads to the differential diagnosis of tremor syndromes. In this context, the unilaterality of the tremor favours the diagnosis of PD or of a dystonic tremor, whereas ET seems to be unlikely due to the asymmetric distribution and character of the tremor and the absence of any family history. The combination of a predominant resting tremor of pill-rolling character and mild bradykinesia, however, narrows down the list to parkinsonian conditions. In this regard, the absence of 'red flags' such as autonomic features, cognitive difficulties, saccadic abnormalities or cerebellar signs (cf. Cases 6–9) renders an atypical form of parkinsonism rather unlikely and eventually leads to the clinical diagnosis of PD. The suggestion of RBD, though neither entirely specific nor present in all PD patients, also supports the diagnosis of an underlying synucleinopathy in this patient.

Investigations and Diagnosis

Whereas a previous brain MRI was completely normal, a DaT-Scan showed reduced bilateral tracer-uptake in the putamen, thus confirming underlying nigrostriatal degeneration. The clinical presentation and the slow progression favour the diagnosis of PD. As there is no diagnostic test for PD, the above-mentioned investigations just support the clinical work-up and are useful in excluding unusual presentations of parkinsonism (such as parenchymal lesions). The final diagnosis of PD, however, is still entirely made on the basis of clinical findings.

Special Remarks

Basically, tremulous and non-tremulous forms of PD are distinguished although recent research suggests that the clinical spectrum in PD may not be restricted to only these two forms. Bradykinesia is the common hallmark in PD and is present in both subtypes whereas other clinical features of parkinsonism including tremor and rigidity are variably present (Movement Disorder Society Clinical Diagnostic Criteria for PD).

Age of onset widely varies, though an onset under the age of 40 is rather uncommon and is most likely to be due to an underlying monogenetic mutation (cf. Table 3.1). A loss of dopaminergic neurons and Lewy bodies pathology are the histological hallmark of PD.

The distribution of these findings is closely related to disease progression. Initially, these changes are present just in the brain stem, olfactory bulb and autonomic system, but subsequently spread to supratentorial regions. In general, the tremulous subtype of PD is thought to have a slower progression rate than the akinetic-rigid subtype.

When making the diagnosis of PD, even by movement disorder specialists there is an error rate of between 10 per cent and 20 per cent. Conditions such as vascular parkinsonism, ET or dystonic tremor or some forms of atypical parkinsonian syndromes may be misdiagnosed as PD. In the context of the tremulous subtype, differentiation from other tremor forms may be challenging particularly when a severe limb tremor interferes with repetitive movement task, thus making it difficult to judge whether there is bradykinesia or not. There might be in fact diagnostic uncertainty in some tremulous patients at the borders of the classification of PD, and motor fluctuations and levodopa-induced dyskinesias are the only reliable clinical features predicting PD pathology.

Suggested Readings

Berardelli A, Wenning GK, Antonini A et al. EFNS/MDS-ES/ENS [corrected] recommendations for the diagnosis of Parkinson's disease. *Eur J Neurol*. 2013;20:16–34.

Hughes AJ, Daniel SE, Kilford L, Lees AJ. Accuracy of clinical diagnosis of idiopathic Parkinson's disease: a clinico-pathological study of 100 cases. J Neurol Neurosurg Psychiatry. 1992;55:181–4.

Postuma RB, Berg D, Stern M et al. MDS clinical diagnostic criteria for Parkinson's disease. *Mov Disord*. 2015;30:1591-601.

Quinn NP, Schneider SA, Schwingenschuh P, Bhatia KP. Tremor – some controversial aspects. *Mov Disord*. 2011;26:18–23.

 Video 1.1

The video sequence shows a 70-year-old patient with left-sided resting tremor. There is also a mild left-sided postural and action tremor. His finger and foot tapping are bradykinetic on his left side with some interruptions of the motor sequences. On his right side, his movements are also irregular with occasional interruptions, but there is no clear fatiguing. His shoulder shrug is reduced on his left. On walking, his arm swing is decreased on his left with rest tremor appearing, while the pattern of his gait is quite normal.

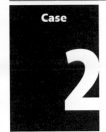

Case

2

Nonmotor Parkinson's Disease

Roberto Erro and Kailash P. Bhatia

Clinical History

A 56-year-old man with a 2-year history of depression and anxiety came to us for the development of a tremor in his right hand in the last 6 months. The tremor was very mild, intermittent and did not bother him in his day-to-day activities, and his main concerns were with regard to his mood. Apart from this, he did not have anything else to report. He denied to have slowed down, and there were no cognitive, autonomic or sleep problems. However, he reported – when asked – that his sense of smell had probably reduced.

Examination

The only abnormal finding on examination was the presence of an intermittent rest tremor of his right hand, most visible when he was mentally distracted. Otherwise, he did not have bradykinesia or rigidity, nor did he look hypomimic. Gait was normal with preserved arm swing. All the remaining neurological examination was unremarkable.

General Remarks

Although rest tremor is highly suggestive of PD, it does not equate PD. In fact, the clinical diagnostic criteria for PD require the presence of bradykinesia plus either rest tremor or rigidity to make the diagnosis. Nevertheless, it is increasingly recognized that PD is not a pure motor disorder and some NMS can predate the onset of motor features by several decades. This is the case for such NMS as depression (as in our case), hyposmia, RBD and constipation. It is hence reasonable to suspect PD in a case like ours, given the combination of rest tremor with depression and possible hyposmia.

Investigations and Diagnosis

A brain MRI was entirely normal, while a DaT-scan turned out to be abnormal with reduced tracer binding in both putamen nuclei (left>right) and relative sparing of the caudate nuclei bilaterally (Figure 2.1). He further underwent a formal smell assessment using the University of Pennsylvania Smell Identification Test, the score of which was 22/40, confirming the presence of hyposmia. This patient has been followed-up for a couple of years during which he developed clear limb bradykinesia, thus making the diagnosis of PD likely.

Special Remarks

It is becoming increasingly clear that PD becomes manifest much before the motor symptoms develop. On research grounds, a proposal to delineate three stages of the disease has been put forth: preclinical, premotor and motor. Such a suggestion relies on the need to identify PD patients earlier, in the face of multiple failed disease modification trials. It has been increasingly recognized that a number of NMS can predate the motor onset of PD and, although no pathological confirmation exists to date, it is well accepted that some of them are highly specific for PD.

The large majority (up to 90 per cent) of PD patients have olfactory dysfunction, including deficits of odor identification, discrimination and threshold. Subjects with hyposmia are estimated to have a relative odd of 5.2 for the development of PD later in life. Similar results were found for depression, and it has been suggested that PD patients had 2.4 times the odds of having a history of depression, as compared to controls, with the first depressive episode preceding the diagnosis of PD by an average of 10 years. Although not specific for PD, the history of RBD has been associated with the development of a neurodegenerative disorder, specifically a synucleinopathy. In the largest prospective series, out of 174 cases with RBD who were followed up for a median of 4 years, up to approximately 38 per cent were eventually diagnosed with a defined neurodegenerative syndrome, with DLB in 29 cases, PD in 22 and MSA in 2. The cumulative risk of developing a neurodegenerative disease was over 90 per cent at 14 years.

Yet, as stated before, there have not yet been pathological confirmation of these results and therefore

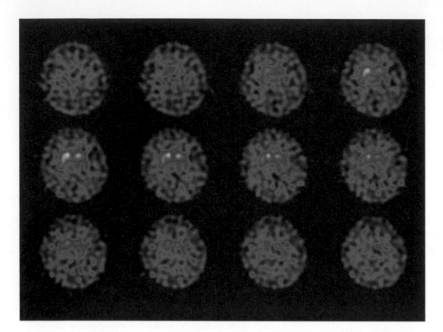

Figure 2.1 DaT-Scan SPECT showing reduced uptake in the posterior putamen (left>right) and relative sparing of the caudate nuclei. A black and white version of this figure will appear in some formats. For the colour version, please refer to the plate section.

a multimodal approach, including imaging, will probably turn more sensitive than the use of any of these NMS, if considered alone. For instance, dopaminergic imaging has been deemed to be abnormal in the premotor stage of the disease, since the first motor symptoms have been estimated to occur after about 80 per cent of striatal and 50 per cent of nigral dopaminergic neurons are lost. Such a multi-modal approach would likely lead to the redefinition of the clinical diagnostic criteria for PD, hopefully allowing an earlier diagnosis.

Suggested Readings

Berg D, Postuma RB, Adler CH, et al. MDS research criteria for prodromal Parkinson's disease. *Mov Disord.* 2015;30:1600–11.

Chahine LM, Stern MB. Characterizing premotor Parkinson's disease: clinical features and objective markers. *Mov Disord Clin Pract.* 2014;1:299–306.

Erro R, Picillo M, Vitale C, et al. Non-motor symptoms in early Parkinson's disease: a 2-year follow-up study on previously untreated patients. *J Neurol Neurosurg Psychiatry.* 2013;84:14–7.

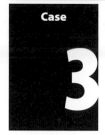

Isolated Lower Limb Dystonia at Onset of Parkin Disease

Roberto Erro and Kailash P. Bhatia

Clinical History

A 47-year-old man of Indian origin, born from non-consanguineous parents and without family history for any neurological disorders, presented with a 2-year history of walking difficulties due to abnormal posturing of his left foot, which was remarkably worse after prolonged exercise. He has also had a couple of falls in which he has tripped forward. The abnormal posturing of his left foot was very mild at onset and could fluctuate, being absent early in the morning or after resting. Because of such marked fluctuations, his symptoms were initially thought to be psychogenic. However, his dystonia became more constant and troublesome during the past 10 months. He also referred to a loss of dexterity in his hands, particularly the right one. Sleep, memory, and mood were reported to be unaffected.

Examination

The only abnormal finding on examination was the presence of dystonia of his left foot (Video 3.1). Such a dystonic posturing was less evident when the patient was asked to walk backwards or with bent knees. There was a doubtful bradykinesia when finger tapping on the right, whereas there was no rigidity and tremor. The remaining neurological examination was normal.

General Remarks

The very first symptom in this patient was the abnormal posturing of his left foot after prolonged exercise, which has been referred to in the literature as PED. PED can be isolated or can be associated with other symptoms. Indeed, the syndromic association of PED with other clinical symptoms/signs can guide investigations to reach the diagnosis. Several disorders can present with PED, including DRD due to *GCH1* mutations, GLUT-1 deficiency syndrome due to mutations in the *SLC2A1* gene, which encodes the glucose transporter type-1, and early onset PD, often due to mutations in the *parkin* gene (Table 3.1). In the former two

(DRD and GLUT-1) the age at onset is usually early in life (within the first two decades), while in our case the onset was later at 45 years of age; there was also the additional complaint about having lost some manual dexterity of his hand. Hence, early onset PD was the most likely diagnosis, despite the absence of clear bradykinesia on examination.

Investigations and Diagnosis

A brain MRI was entirely normal, while a DaT-Scan turned out to be abnormal with reduced tracer binding in both putamen nuclei and relative sparing of the caudate nuclei bilaterally. Given the young age at onset, further genetic testing for PD genes was pursued, and the patient was found to be compound heterozygous for the c.C1000T mutation in exon 9 and an exon 2 deletion in the *parkin* gene.

Special Remarks

Parkinsonism due to mutations in the *parkin* gene, also referred to as PARK2, is an autosomal recessive genetic entity, typically presenting with young-onset (<40 years) parkinsonism, and/or predominant lower limb dystonia, which can be paroxysmal in the earliest stage. A dramatic response to L-dopa and a benign and slow progression are usually seen, even though parkin patients can have early L-dopa-induced dyskinesia. While young age of onset is undoubtedly the best clinical indicator of such a genetic disorder, Parkin disease accounting for up to 15 per cent of early onset sporadic PD patients, the condition has also been occasionally reported in patients with onset above the age of 50 years. Additional symptoms and signs that increase the likelihood of a positive gene test are brisk reflexes, early autonomic dysfunction, peripheral neuropathy and marked psychiatric features, including severe anxiety and obsessive-compulsive symptoms. In some cases, however, the phenotype is limited to isolated lower limb dystonia, and differentiating between DRD and

Table 3.1 PARK-Designated PD-Related Loci*

Locus	Chromosome	Gene	Inheritance	Phenotype
PARK1/PARK4	4q21	SNCA	AD	EOPD with early dementia
PARK2	6q25.2-q27	Parkin	AR	EOPD
PARK3 (unconfirmed)	2p13	Unknown	AD	Classical PD
PARK5 (unconfirmed)	4p13	UCLH1	Unclear	Classical PD
PARK6	1p36	PINK1	AR	EOPD
PARK7	1p36	DJ-1	AR	EOPD
PARK8	12q12	LRRK2	AD	Classical PD
PARK9	1p36	ATP13A2	AR	Juvenile PD, pyramidal sign, dementia, possible iron accumulation on imaging
PARK10 (unconfirmed)	1p32	Unknown	Risk factor	Late onset parkinsonism
PARK11	2q37	Unknown	Risk factor	Late onset parkinsonism
PARK12 (unconfirmed)	Xq21-25	Unknown	X-linked	Late onset parkinsonism
PARK13 (unconfirmed)	2p12	HTRA2	AD or risk factor	Late onset parkinsonism
PARK14	22q12-q13	PLA2G6	AR	Dystonia-parkinsonism, (late) iron accumulation on imaging
PARK15	22q12-q13	FBXO7	AR	Juvenile parkinsonism and pyramidal signs
PARK16 (unconfirmed)	1q32	Unknown	Risk factor	Late onset parkinsonism
PARK17	16q11.2	VPS3A	AD	Classical PD
PARK18 (unconfirmed)	3q27.1	EIF4G1	AD	Classical PD
PARK19	1p31.3	DNAJC6	AR	Juvenile parkinsonism with pyramidal signs, dystonia, seizures and mental retardation
PARK20	21q22.11	SYNJ1	AR	Juvenile parkinsonism with rapid progression and severe L-dopa dyskinesias, possible seizures

* Note that other two genes, namely *TMEM230* and *CHCHD2*, transmitted in an AD fashion, have been associated with adult onset typical PD but they have not been confirmed yet or have not been assigned any PARK-number.
Abb.: AD: autosomal dominant; AR: autosomal recessive; EOPD: early onset Parkinson disease.
Source: Modified from Sheerin UM, Houlden H, Wood NW. Advances in the genetics of Parkinson's disease: a guide for the clinician. *Mov Disord Clin Pract*. 2014;1:3–13.

a DRD-like presentation of parkin disease can be difficult. Additional investigations including cerebrospinal fluid (CSF) examination and/or DaT-Scan (cf. Case 20) are therefore required.

Suggested Readings

Elia AE, Del Sorbo F, Romito LM, Barzaghi C, Garavaglia B, Albanese A. Isolated limb dystonia as presenting feature of Parkin disease. *J Neurol Neurosurg Psychiatry*. 2014;85:827–8.

Erro R, Stamelou M, Ganos C, et al. The clinical syndrome of paroxysmal exercise-induced dystonia: diagnostic outcomes and an algorithm. *Mov Disord Clin Pract*. 2014;1:57–61.

Khan NL, Graham E, Critchley P, et al. Parkin disease: a phenotypic study of a large case series. *Brain*. 2003;126:1279–92.

 Video 3.1

Abnormal posturing of the right foot, which is turned inwards. The dystonic posturing improves when the patient walks backwards or with his knees flexed.

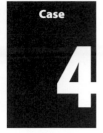

Case

4

Parkinson's Disease Associated with *SNCA* Mutations

Leonidas Stefanis and Maria Stamelou

Clinical History

This 49-year-old woman of Greek origin first noticed a rest tremor of her left arm at the age of 46 years. She also noticed moderate depressive symptoms and excessive fatigue. Her symptoms were progressive, and over the next 2 years she developed stiffness more on the left and mild gait problems. She was diagnosed with PD and was prescribed rasagiline 1 mg/day and ropinirole up to 6 mg/day, and her motor symptoms improved. Over the next year there was a need to increase ropinirole (up to 12 mg/day) as the patient was experiencing unsteadiness increasingly, mostly with the left foot, which she felt she was dragging, and also because of the worsening of her tremor. Three years after disease onset she required a further increase of ropinirole and also a small dose of levodopa (150 mg/day), as her motor symptoms progressed. Regarding her family history, her father was diagnosed with PD in his fifties, developed dementia rapidly, and died in his sixties; her paternal aunt was also diagnosed with PD later in life.

Examination

On examination (see Video 4.1) it was found that she had broken smooth pursuit and slightly slow saccades. She had mild hypomimia and no dysarthria. There was asymmetrical mild bradykinesia and rigidity on upper and lower limbs more on the left, as well as a rest and kinetic tremor more on left arm and leg. There was reduced arm swing on the left when walking, and a slight dragging of the left foot upon excessive tiredness. There was no postural instability.

General Remarks

The clinical signs are compatible with sporadic PD. However, the early age of onset and the positive family history would suggest a genetic cause of the patient's symptoms. Because of the Greek origin of the patient, and the apparent autosomal dominant mode of inheritance, a mutation in the alpha-synuclein (*SNCA*) gene should be suspected (cf. Table 3.1).

Investigations and Diagnosis

A brain MRI scan was normal. A DaT-Scan was severely abnormal more on the right, corresponding to the clinical picture. Autonomic function tests showed a mild orthostatic hypotension and a mild urinary urgency. Neuropsychiatric assessment showed no cognitive dysfunction. DNA testing confirmed the G209A missense mutation in the *SNCA* gene.

Special Remarks

The G209A missense mutation in the *SNCA* gene leading to a p.A53T substitution is associated with autosomal dominant PD and has been originally described in families of Greek or Italian origin. Cognitive decline has been reported in many affected individuals carrying the p.A53T mutation, and the phenotype is usually more consistent with PD dementia or Lewy body dementia. Although generally it is thought that patients carrying this mutation are of very young onset and severely impaired, there is large phenotypic variability both in terms of age of onset, progression and associated features. Thus, even in an otherwise typical PD, if there is family history compatible with autosomal dominant inheritance, and in particular if the patient is of Greek or Italian origin, one should screen for mutations in the *SNCA* gene.

Suggested Readings

Papadimitriou D, Antonelou R, Miligkos M, et al. Motor and non-motor features of carriers of the p.A53T alpha-synuclein mutation: a longitudinal study. Mov Disord, 2016.;31:1226–30.

Ricciardi L, Petrucci S, Di Giuda D, et al. The Contursi family 20 years later: intrafamilial phenotypic variability of the SNCA p.A53T mutation. *Mov Disord*. 2016;31:257–8.

Video 4.1

Left-sided rest tremor of the upper and lower limb. Bradykinesia on finger tapping is shown on the left. Gait is reasonably long stepped, but arm swing is reduced.

PSP: Steele-Richardson-Olszewski Syndrome

Pedro Barbosa, Helen Ling, Eduardo de Pablo-Fernandez,
Janice Holton, and Thomas Warner

Clinical History

A 60-year-old male was referred to a neurologist because his family noticed that he had developed flat affect and he also had started driving erratically. A few months after these symptoms he developed a robotic gait with staring, speech changes, and an abnormal posture on his left hand.

Approximately 9 months later he started falling particularly backwards and sideways. Subsequently he developed slow speech abnormalities and hypophonia, as well as cervical dystonia and urinary incontinence. He was wheelchair bound after 5 years after the first symptoms started and died 2 years later of aspiration pneumonia, after 7 years of disease.

Examination

Initially, there was facial hypomimia without any other parkinsonian signs, followed by slow vertical saccades and a marked reduction in blinking frequency. In the following assessments he developed speech problems, bilateral palmomental reflex, neck rigidity, square wave jerks, and an involuntary posture of left hand with extension of two fingers. Eventually, a vertical supranuclear gaze palsy became evident along with the classic growling speech and hypophonia and the emergence of the procerus sign (Video 5.1).

General Remarks

This patient presented with a parkinsonian syndrome with some atypical features, including eye movement abnormalities, a tendency to fall backwards, and a relatively rapid progression leading to death within 7 years, which are all against the diagnosis of PD. Classically, patients have eye movement abnormalities, particularly vertical supranuclear gaze palsy (Richardson's syndrome) with downward gaze abnormalities. Other ocular abnormalities are also common in PSP, and early features preceding vertical supranuclear palsy include square wave jerks and slowing of vertical saccades.

The detection of the 'round the houses' sign, an early manifestation of slow vertical saccades, may be useful in clinching the diagnosis of PSP in the early disease.

Early falls is a common feature in PSP and the clinical criteria of probable PSP-RS requires unprovoked falls to occur within 12 months of disease onset. However, many pathologically confirmed PSP patients experience their first fall after one year of symptoms onset. The growling speech is a classic feature incorporating component of dysarthria, hypophonia, and possible spasticity. Dystonia can also be present in PSP patients, and the most common sites are limbs, eyelids, and axial muscles. Overlapped clinical features reminiscent of corticobasal syndrome are not uncommon in patients with a PSP-like syndrome such as unilateral dystonia and ideomotor apraxia of the upper limb and limb levitation.

Investigations

Imaging of the dopamine transporter system was performed revealing reduced uptake of transporter in the lenticular nuclei. MRI of the brain showed subtle volume loss of the midbrain and superior colliculi, as well as mild degree of cortical atrophy.

Pathology and Diagnosis

On autopsy, macroscopic findings included mild atrophy of the frontal lobe, prominent atrophy of the subthalamic nucleus, marked pallor of the substantia nigra and possibly locus coeruleus, reduction in height of the tegmentum in the midbrain and pons, atrophy of the superior cerebellar peduncle, and dentate nucleus in the cerebellum. At histological examination (Figure 5.1), prominent tau pathology involving both neurons and glial cells with frequent neurofibrillary tangles, pre-tangles, neuropil threads, coiled bodies, and tufted astrocytes in neocortical regions, deep grey nuclei, brain stem, and cerebellum were observed, thus confirming the diagnosis of PSP.

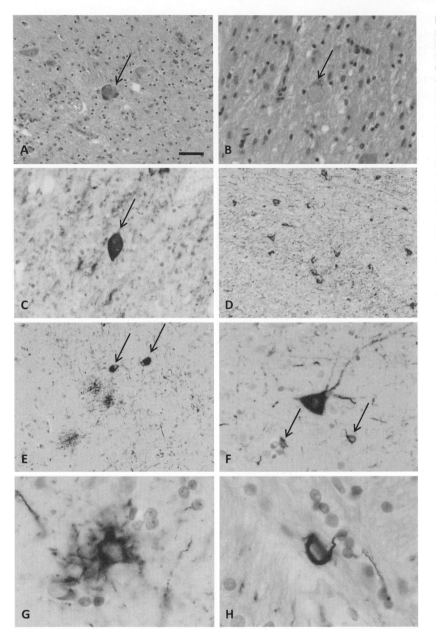

Figure 5.1 Histological examination showed neuropathological changes of progressive supranuclear palsy. In the substantia nigra there was moderate loss of dopaminergic pigmented neurons, and some residual neurons contained basophilic neurofibrillary tangles (A, arrow indicates a neuron with a neurofibrillary tangle). In the subthalamic nucleus there was gliosis and neuronal loss with neurofibrillary tangles in several surviving neurons (B, arrow indicates a neuron containing a neurofibrillary tangle), confirmed by positive staining using tau immunohistochemistry (C, arrow). In the cerebellar white matter there were numerous coiled bodies and threads (D). Tau positive structures in the frontal cortex (E and F) included neurofibrillary tangles (E, arrows) and tufted astrocytes (E) while higher magnification revealed several coiled bodies (F, arrows). In the caudate nucleus, typical tufted astrocytes were found (G) and there were numerous coiled bodies in the internal capsule (H).
(Bar in A represents 50 μm in A, D, & E; 25 μm in B, C, & F; 10 μm in G & H. Haematoxylin and eosin: A & B. Tau immunohistochemistry: C–H.) A black and white version of this figure will appear in some formats. For the colour version, please refer to the plate section.

Special Remarks

PSP is more common in men and its prevalence ranges from 1 to 6.5 cases per 100,000 population.

The clinical diagnosis of PSP relies on accurate history taking, clinical examination including careful eye movement examination, and midbrain atrophy on neuroimaging leading to the classic 'Hummingbird sign' (Figure 5.2). The clinical diagnosis accuracy is between 70 and 80 per cent and with the absence of a biomarker; the diagnosis of PSP can only be confirmed at post-mortem including the finding of tufted astrocytes, the pathognomonic histological hallmark, in a typical distribution.

The increasingly recognized phenotypic variability of PSP (cf. Case 6) may account for the low sensitivity of the current clinical criteria for the diagnosis of PSP and for the relatively high rate of misdiagnosis. Although some patients may experience transient symptomatic

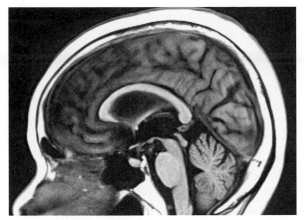

Figure 5.2 Sagittal T1-weighted image showing severe midbrain atrophy that results in a characteristic profile of the brainstem (the 'hummingbird sign') in which the preserved pons forms the body of the bird, and the atrophic midbrain the head, with beak extending anteriorly towards the optic chiasm.

improvement with dopaminergic therapy and with the use of Amantadine, currently, no treatment is available to PSP. Mean survival after disease onset can vary from 5.6 to 7 years, and the majority of patients die from respiratory-related causes.

Suggested Readings

Hauw JJ, Daniel SE, Dickson D, et al. Preliminary NINDS neuropathologic criteria for Steele-Richardson-Olszewski syndrome (progressive supranuclear palsy). *Neurology*. 1994;44:2015–19.

Litvan I, Agid Y, Jankovic J, et al. Accuracy of clinical criteria for the diagnosis of progressive supranuclear palsy (Steele-Richardson-Olszewski syndrome). *Neurology*. 1996;46:922–30.

Papapetropoulos S, Gonzalez J, Mash DC. Natural history of progressive supranuclear palsy: a clinicopathologic study from a population of brain donors. *Eur Neurol*. 2005;54:1–9.

  Video 5.1

Segment 1: gait showing broad base with instability and backwards fall after turning 180 degrees; Segment 2: postural instability; Segment 3: two years later there is marked worsening of gait; Segment 4: restriction of downward gaze; Segment 5: bradykinesia; Segment 6: speech abnormalities.

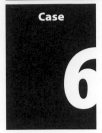

Case

PSP-Parkinsonism

Pedro Barbosa, Helen Ling, Eduardo de Pablo-Fernandez, Janice Holton, and Thomas Warner

Clinical History

A 60-year-old male developed progressive difficulty with walking, particularly with freezing, which lead to frequent falls. Three years later he developed speech abnormalities with hoarseness of voice and hypophonia, and difficulties doing up buttons.

A few months later he developed eye movement abnormalities, particularly restriction of downward gaze and periods of involuntary closure of his eyes. Levodopa was prescribed with moderate improvement of his symptoms.

The disease progressed relentlessly and 9 years after the onset of the first symptoms he was having daily backward falls and developed complete restriction of vertical gaze. He was still having moderate benefit from levodopa with a daily dose of approximately 450 mg per day.

He died at 70 years old from respiratory failure secondary to aspiration pneumonia, 10 years after disease onset.

Examination

Neurological examination 3 years after the onset of the first symptoms showed unsteady gait and axial rigidity. Cranial nerve examination showed mild limitation of vertical eye movement and apraxia of eyelid opening. There was asymmetrical limb rigidity with cogwheeling, worse on the right side and upper limb bradykinesia. Initially there was an upper limb rest and postural tremor, which developed an intention component over time. Repetitive finger tapping was of small amplitude and good speed without decrement (Video 6.1).

As the disease progressed, he developed complete restriction of voluntary gaze and partial restriction of horizontal gaze (approximately 50 per cent) and a marked worsening of the eye-lid apraxia, remaining approximately 80 per cent of the time with his eyes closed involuntarily. The applause sign was evident only in the last years of disease, when the patient exhibited a positive response with 8 claps.

General Remarks

The most common diagnosis in patients presenting with levodopa responsive asymmetrical parkinsonism is PD. However, early postural instability in this patient was a clinical red flag and would suggest a diagnosis of PSP. PSP-RS (cf. Case 5) and PSP-P are the two main phenotypic presentation of PSP. PSP-P is a more benign form, with a more protracted course and clinical features similar to PD including moderate response to levodopa and unilateral hand tremor which is often more jerky in nature and more prominent on action. In more advanced stages, patients with PSP-P usually, but not always, begin to manifest clinical symptoms and signs more typical of Richardson's syndrome including vertical supranuclear gaze palsy.

Moreover, patients with PSP irrespective of phenotype have a distinct finger-tapping pattern without decrement or fatigue, unlike the criteria-defined bradykinesia observed in patients with PD. This simple bedside test can assist clinicians to distinguish PSP-P from PD. The applause sign is an indicator of frontal disinhibition and is commonly abnormal in PSP.

Investigations

An MRI of his brain, performed 6 years after disease onset, showed mild small vessel disease and a reduced midbrain volume.

Pathology and Diagnosis

Pathological examination (Figure 6.1) demonstrated marked pallor of the substantia nigra and locus coeruleus, mild reduction in the height of the tegmentum of the midbrain and pons, severe atrophy and gliosis of the subthalamic nucleus, mild atrophy of the globus pallidus and frontal cortex, mild neuronal loss and gliosis in the dentate nucleus. Tau immunohistochemistry revealed frequent tufted astrocytes, sparse

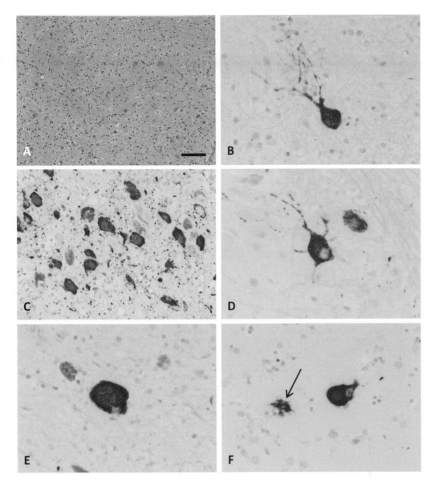

Figure 6.1 Histological examination confirmed neuronal and glial tau pathology with a distribution and type typical of progressive supranuclear palsy. In the dentate nucleus there was gliosis and mild loss of neurons (A), a number of the remaining neurons contained tau immunoreactive neurofibrillary tangles (B). The locus coeruleus was well preserved but contained numerous neurofibrillary tangles (C) and these were also present in modest numbers in the pontine nuclei (D). The substantia nigra showed severe loss of pigmented neurons with neurofibrillary tangles in several remaining neurons (E). There were scattered neurofibrillary tangles and tufted astrocytes (arrow) in the caudate nucleus (F).

(Bar in A represents 100 μm in A; 50 μm in C; 25 μm in B, D, E, & F. Haematoxylin and eosin: A. Tau immunohistochemistry: B – F.) A black and white version of this figure will appear in some formats. For the colour version, please refer to the plate section.

neurofibrillary tangles and neuropil threads in the caudate nucleus. These features were consistent with the diagnosis of PSP.

Special Remarks

In a clinicopathological study of PSP, 32 per cent of patients with the PSP-P phenotype had clinical features of asymmetric rest tremor at onset and an initial response to treatment with levodopa. Patients with PSP-P have a longer survival than those with PSP-RS and tend to experience some level of improvement in rigidity and bradykinesia with levodopa treatment, even though the response may not sustain in more advanced stages. Thus, the distinction from PD may be impossible early in the disease but careful examination of eye movements may reveal subtle abnormal features such as square wave jerks or slowing of vertical saccades. However, after some years into the disease, the majority of PSP-P patients would develop the full-blown phenotype of Richardson's syndrome including vertical supranuclear gaze palsy and prominent postural instability.

Differences in the distribution of neuronal loss and tau pathology have been shown to correlate with the different clinical phenotypes of PSP. Patients with PSP-P tend to exhibit less severe and more restricted tau pathology, affecting mainly the subthalamic nucleus, substantia nigra, and internal globus pallidus when compared to PSP-RS.

Suggested Readings

Ling H, Massey LA, Lees AJ, Brown P, Day BL. Hypokinesia without decrement distinguishes progressive supranuclear palsy from Parkinson's disease. *Brain*. 2012;135:1141–53.

Williams DR, Lees AJ. Progressive supranuclear palsy: clinicopathological concepts and diagnostic challenges. *Lancet Neurology*. 2009;8:270–9.

Williams DR, de Silva R, Paviour DC, et al. Characteristics of two distinct clinical phenotypes in pathologically proven progressive supranuclear palsy: Richardson's syndrome and PSP-parkinsonism. *Brain.* 2005;128:1247–58.

 Video 6.1

Finger-tapping manoeuvre showing absence of decrement and bradykinesia.

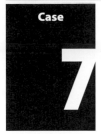

Case 7

Corticobasal Degeneration

Eduardo de Pablo-Fernandez, Helen Ling, Pedro Barbosa,
Tamas Revesz, and Thomas Warner

Clinical History

A 70-year-old man presented with difficulties using his right arm when performing fine movements and also complex motor tasks. Symptoms gradually progressed and his right arm became functionally useless. A few years later, he developed gait difficulties with falls and cognitive deterioration with expressive dysphasia and symptoms of executive dysfunction, such as difficulties planning activities, performing complex motor tasks, and poor attention. Motor symptoms did not respond to L-dopa. His right arm developed a flexed posture with clawing of his hand. His mobility was impaired requiring use of a wheelchair and he developed marked cognitive deterioration. He died 8 years after symptom onset.

Examination

Six years after symptom onset, bedside cognitive examination showed expressive dysphasia with preserved comprehension, right-sided sensory inattention, ideomotor apraxia, and cortical sensory loss with astereognosis and agraphaesthesia. Applause sign was negative.

Ocular saccade initiation was delayed with associated head thrusts (Video 7.1). There was no weakness, and reflexes were present and symmetrical. He had stimulus sensitive myoclonus involving both arms. Severe bradykinesia and cogwheel rigidity was present in the right arm, which was held in a flexed dystonic posture. His gait was unsteady, dragging the right leg, but his postural reflexes were preserved.

General Remarks

The core clinical features in this patient are a progressive, asymmetrical, L-dopa unresponsive parkinsonism with other additional motor symptoms (dystonia, myoclonus) in combination with cortical signs including parietal dysfunction, dysphasia, and cortical sensory loss. This combination of symptoms, referred as CBS, is the classic clinical phenotype of CBD. However, several clinicopathological series have demonstrated that CBS can be associated with multiple other pathologies in addition to CBD, most commonly PSP and AD, followed by other forms of FTLD. As a result, the term CBS is now used to describe the clinical syndrome during life (as in this case), while CBD is applied to the pathological condition requiring histopathological confirmation.

Investigations

Brain MRI showed generalized cortical atrophy with focal volume loss involving the superior parietal and frontal lobes more marked on the left (Figure 7.1). A DaT-Scan showed bilateral reduction of tracer uptake consistent with nigrostriatal dopaminergic degeneration. A formal neuropsychological examination demonstrated marked cognitive impairment involving mainly cortical and subcortical areas of the dominant fronto-parietal lobes with non-fluent aphasia, acalculia, dyspraxia, executive dysfunction, and slow information processing speed.

Pathology and Diagnosis

A postmortem examination was performed. On macroscopic examination there was mild atrophy of the frontal and anterior parietal lobes in a parasagittal distribution with associated pallor of the substantia nigra. Histopathological examination (Figure 7.2) demonstrated widespread tau-positive lesions affecting both neurons (neuronal threads) and glial cells (astrocytic plaques). Neuronal loss and gliosis was noted in the substantia nigra and cortical areas with a few ballooned neurons. These findings were consistent with the diagnosis of CBD.

Special Remarks

CBS is considered the classic presentation of CBD but it is now well accepted that other phenotypes are associated with CBD pathology including PSP-RS,

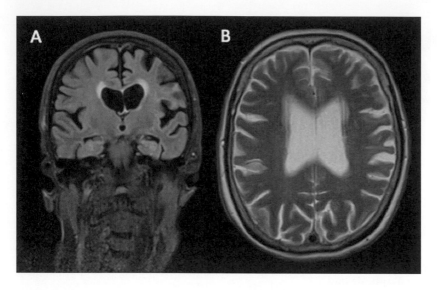

Figure 7.1 Coronal FLAIR (A) and axial T2-weighted (B) images showing asymmetric cortical atrophy more prominent in the left perirolandic gyri, superior parietal, and frontal lobes.

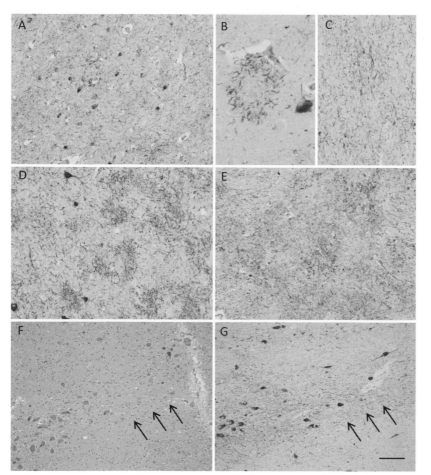

Figure 7.2 Tau immunohistochemistry demonstrates numerous pretangles, neurofibrillary tangles, and neuropil threads in the prefrontal cortex (A). Astrocytic plaques, which are one of the diagnostic criteria of corticobasal degeneration, were readily found in cerebral cortices and subcortical nuclei in this case (B). Tau-positive neurites and threads were numerous in the subcortical white matter (C). The tau pathology with numerous neuropil threads and astrocytic plaques was severe in both the amygdala (D) and caudate nucleus (E). The loss of neuromelaning-containing neurons (arrows) was of moderate degree in the pars compacta of the substantia nigra (F), but most of the remaining neurons contained either pretangles or neurofibrillary tangles (G).

(Bar on G represents 160 microns on F and G, 80 microns on A, C-E, and 40 microns on B. A-E and G: tau immunohistochemistry (AT8 antibody); F: haematoxylin and eosin stain.) A black and white version of this figure will appear in some formats. For the colour version, please refer to the plate section.

behavioural, and aphasic variants of FTLD among other neurodegenerative conditions. These multiple phenotypes demonstrate that CBD should be considered as a continuum combining cognitive deficits and movement disorders, crossing the classic division between movement and cognition domains. The antemortem prediction of pathologies underlying CBS on clinical grounds is difficult and no signs can differentiate with certainty these conditions. The presence of delayed horizontal saccades with normal velocity and cortical sensory loss reflecting parietal involvement might predict CBD pathology as opposed to slow vertical saccades and more frontal pattern of cognitive impairment more consistent with PSP. The course of the symptoms might be useful in the differential diagnoses. Prion disease, progranulin, *C9ORF72* mutations, and FTLD-FUS should be considered in cases with rapid clinical progression, cerebrovascular disease when there is an acute onset with a static course, while slow progression and sustained L dopa response of the symptoms is more consistent with PD. Established amyloid scan and CSF biomarkers are useful in recognizing Alzheimer's disease pathology (AD-CBS).

Owing to the clinicopathological heterogeneity, diagnostic criteria incorporating the increasing number of pathological aetiologies have been proposed to improve the diagnostic accuracy in life, which remains the main challenge of this complex neurodegenerative disorder.

Suggested Readings

Armstrong MJ, Litvan I, Lang AE, et al. Criteria for the diagnosis of corticobasal degeneration. *Neurology*. 2013;80:496–503.

Kouri N, Whitwell JL, Josephs KA, et al. Corticobasal degeneration: a pathologically distinct 4R tauopathy. *Nat Rev Neurol*. 2011;7:263–72.

Ling H, O'Sullivan S, Holton JL, et al. Does corticobasal degeneration exist? A clinicopathological re-evaluation. *Brain*. 2010;133:2045–57.

Mathew R, Bak TH, Hodges JR. Diagnostic criteria for corticobasal syndrome: a comparative study. *J Neurol Neurosurg Psychiatry*. 2012;8:400–5.

 Video 7.1

Segment 1: delayed ocular saccades with associated head thrusts; Segment 2: apraxic pattern of gait; Segment 3: oro-buccal and limb apraxia, action myoclonus and magnetism of the left arm.

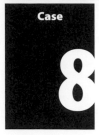

MSA – Parkinsonian Variant

Eduardo de Pablo-Fernandez, Helen Ling, Pedro Barbosa,
Janice Holton, and Thomas Warner

Clinical History

A 63-year-old woman presented with episodes of urinary incontinence and incomplete bladder emptying. These symptoms progressed and she developed recurrent urinary infections, eventually requiring intermittent self-catheterization and subsequently a permanent suprapubic catheter. At age 67 she noticed progressive gait difficulties, loss of hand dexterity when performing fine movements, and a postural tremor. Her balance deteriorated and she had repeated falls requiring a walker to mobilize. In addition, she developed nonmotor symptoms with constipation, sleep fragmentation, drooling, and dysarthria. There were no changes in the sense of smell, orthostatic symptoms, or symptoms of RBD. Her condition did not improve with L-dopa and she became reliant on a wheelchair due to progressive deterioration of her mobility. She died 5 years after symptom onset.

Examination

Examination at age 68 (Video 8.1) showed marked facial hypomimia, reduced blink rate, dysarthria, and right torticollis. She had a gaze-evoked nystagmus in horizontal gaze. No orofacial dyskinesias were noted. In the upper limbs there was symmetrical moderate bradykinesia with rigidity and a postural tremor. No polyminimyoclonus were noted. Reflexes were brisk and both plantar responses were extensor. There was mild bilateral limb ataxia on finger–nose test.

General Remarks

The combination of autonomic failure, parkinsonism, and ataxia in this patient pointed to the diagnosis of MSA. Based on the predominant motor feature at presentation there are two MSA clinical subtypes, a parkinsonian (MSA-P) and a cerebellar variant (MSA-C, cf. Case 62), which correlate with the presence of

SND or OPC atrophy on imaging and neuropathology. Given the predominant parkinsonian signs she was diagnosed with MSA-P in life which was confirmed on post-mortem examination.

Investigations

A brain MRI showed putaminal atrophy and hyperintensity of the pons consistent with 'hot cross bun' sign (Figure 8.1). Autonomic function test demonstrated cardiovascular autonomic failure with blocked Valsalva, reduced heart rate variability, orthostatic hypotension on head up-tilt, and absence of nocturnal circadian dip in blood pressure.

Pathology and Diagnosis

A post-mortem examination was performed. Macroscopic examination showed atrophy and discolouration of the posterior part of the putamen and marked pallor of the substantia nigra. Mild cerebellar atrophy was also noted.

Histopathological examination (Figure 8.2) showed moderate gliosis and cell loss involving the dorsal part of the putamen with severe loss of pigmented neurons in the substantia nigra. Milder neuronal loss was also noted involving the locus coeruleus, pontine base, and cerebellum. Immunohistochemistry showed widespread α-synuclein positive glial cytoplasmic inclusions in oligodendrocytes, the MSA pathological hallmark. These findings were consistent with the pathological diagnoses of MSA with predominant SND changes.

Special Remarks

MSA-P is the most prevalent form of MSA in Western countries and usually presents with asymmetrical parkinsonism and dysautonomia. Early clinical diagnosis is often challenging though the presence of early postural instability, a jerky myoclonic postural tremor,

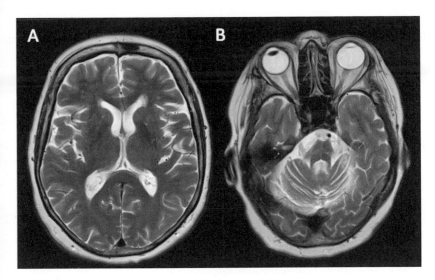

Figure 8.1 Axial T2 weighted images showing putaminal atrophy (A) and signal changes in the pons ('hot cross bun' sign) with marked infratentorial volume loss (B).

poor and transient response to L-dopa (which can trigger orofacial dyskinesias), and rapid progression with early immobility are helpful clinical clues to differentiate it from PD with autonomic failure. Recent evidence suggests that non-motor features such as autonomic failure, sleep disorders, and respiratory problems might precede the development of the classic motor features of MSA by several years. In the case presented here, she developed urinary symptoms a few years before any motor impairment. Recognition of these symptoms can help to make an early and accurate clinical diagnosis and has therapeutic implications as early autonomic dysfunction and nocturnal respiratory problems have been associated with poor prognosis. Moreover, some of these symptoms are present in almost all MSA patients, such as erectile dysfunction in men and urinary incontinence in women, and their absence should be considered as red flags to revise the diagnosis.

Neuroimaging can be helpful in the differential diagnosis, though the described putaminal and pontine abnormalities are not specific and are often only present in advanced stages when the clinical diagnosis is more certain. Consensus criteria have been developed but a definite diagnosis requires histopathological confirmation.

Suggested Readings

Gilman S, Wenning GK, Low PA, et al. Second consensus statement on the diagnosis of multiple system atrophy. *Neurology.* 2008;71:670–6.

Jecmenica-Lukic M, Poewe W, Tolosa E, Wenning GK. Premotor signs and symptoms of multiple system atrophy. *Lancet Neurol.* 2012;11:361–8.

Ozawa T, Paviour D, Quinn NP, et al. The spectrum of pathological involvement of the striatonigral and olivopontocerebellar systems in multiple system atrophy: clinicopathological correlations. *Brain.* 2004;127:2657–71.

Petrovic IN, Ling H, Asi Y, et al. Multiple system atrophy-parkinsonism with slow progression and prolonged survival: a diagnostic catch. *Movement Disorders.* 2012;27:1186–90.

Stefanova N, Bücke P, Duerr S, Wenning GK. Multiple system atrophy: an update. *Lancet Neurol.* 2009;8:1172–8.

   Video 8.1

Segment 1: broken pursuit eye movements with associated gaze-evoked nystagmus and dysmetric saccades; Segment 2: bilateral bradykinesia; Segment 3: limb ataxia with dysmetria and dysdiadochokinesia.

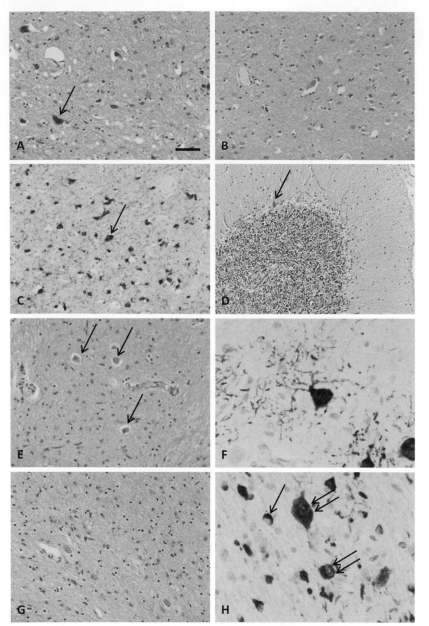

Figure 8.2 Histological examination showed typical features of multiple system atrophy with involvement of striatonigral and olivopontocerebellar regions. There was marked loss of pigmented neurons in the substantia nigra with scattered clusters of neuromelanin in the neuropil (A, arrow indicates a residual pigmented neuron). In the putamen there was moderate neuronal loss (B) and α-synuclein immunohistochemistry demonstrated frequent neuronal cytoplasmic inclusions (arrow) and glial cytoplasmic inclusions (C). Only sparse residual Purkinje cells were present in the cerebellum (D, arrow). The inferior olivary nucleus was gliotic with moderate neuronal loss (E, arrows indicate residual neurons) and many residual neurons contained neuronal cytoplasmic inclusions (F). There was also moderate loss of neurons in the pontine nuclei (G) where there were frequent glial cytoplasmic inclusions (arrow), and neurons often contained both cytoplasmic and nuclear inclusions (double arrow) (H).

(Bar in A represents 100 µm in D; 50 µm in A, B, C, E, & G; 25 µm in F & H. Haematoxylin and eosin: A, B, D, E & G. α-Synuclein immunohistochemistry: C, F, & H.) A black and white version of this figure will appear in some formats. For the colour version, please refer to the plate section.

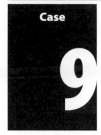

Case

9 Prominent Freezing of Gait and Speech Disturbances Due to Fahr Disease

Roberto Erro and Kailash P. Bhatia

Clinical History

This 57-year-old patient with no relevant family history noted difficulty in writing and walking with associated falls by the age of 53. Shortly after, he developed stuttering (which he never had), erectile dysfunction, and urinary urgency. Symptoms were progressive and he was most affected by his speech and walking difficulties. There were no other complaints and, on specific questioning, he denied symptoms of orthostatic hypotension, sleep disturbances, hallucinations, and/or memory problems.

Examination

On examination, it was found that he had a hypomimic face with frontalis overactivity. The range of his eye movements was full, but the horizontal saccades were hypometric and smooth pursuit movements were broken. There was a marked stammer and a tendency to echolalia, with his speech tending to be 'festinant'. There was a decreased shoulder shrug, while in the upper limbs he had bilateral bradykinesia as well as rigidity with the left arm being affected more than the right. He also showed a jerky postural tremor of the upper limbs. There was some increase in the axial tone but his posture was normal. He had FOG with initiation failure as well as difficulty on turning (Video 9.1). On the pull test he tended to festinate backwards. Moreover, there was a prominent grasp reflex and he tended to mildly perseverate. The remaining neurological examination was normal, apart from the deep tendon reflexes, which were brisk in all limbs.

General Remarks

Although the combination of parkinsonian signs with possible authonomic dysfunction would raise the suspicion of an atypical parkinsonian syndrome, namely MSA (cf. Case 8), there are in this case other features that would not fit in easily with this diagnosis. Specifically, the prominent FOG is not classically seen in patients with MSA and is instead more commonly seen in patients with PSP. On the contrary, the eye movement abnormalities as well as the autonomic dysfunction would not be characteristic of PSP. The prominent 'lower-body' involvement along with the speech disturbances could instead raise the suspicion of vascular parkinsonism. The latter can in fact produce such a phenotype with marked walking difficulties (also referred to as 'high-level gait disorder') when the vascular load is strategically located in the basal ganglia and subcortical frontal areas. Following the same rationale, any kind of lesions occurring in such areas might produce a similar phenotype.

Investigations and Diagnosis

Standard MRI sequences did not reveal major changes attributable to vascular disease, while gradient echo sequences showed marked and diffuse subcortical and gyral areas of susceptibility in both cerebral hemispheres with symmetrical involvement of the basal ganglia and thalami, cerebellar dentate nuclei, and central pons (Figure 9.1). A subsequent CT scan proved that such areas of susceptibility were due to extensive calcifications (Figure 9.2). Biochemical investigations, including serum calcium, phosphorus, magnesium, alkaline phosphatase, calcitonin and parathyroid hormone, as well as genetic testing for *SLC20A2*, *PDGFRB*, and *PDGF-B* mutations yielded normal results. Hence, the patient was diagnosed with PFBC (formerly known as Fahr disease), even in the absence of family history.

Special Remarks

Fahr disease, now termed PFBC, is a rare disorder, which is characterized by abnormal calcium depositions in the brain, typically in the basal ganglia and cerebellum, particularly the dentate nuclei. It is an inherited disorder and, thus, it is differentiated from Fahr syndrome, where abnormal brain calcifications may be secondary to systemic disorders affecting calcium homeostasis such as hypoparathyroidism.

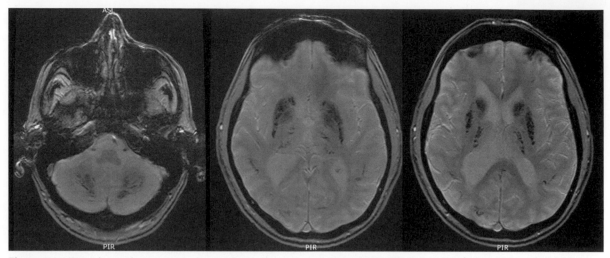

Figure 9.1 MRI gradient-echo sequences showing marked areas of susceptibility with symmetrical involvement of the basal ganglia, thalami, and cerebellar dentate nuclei.

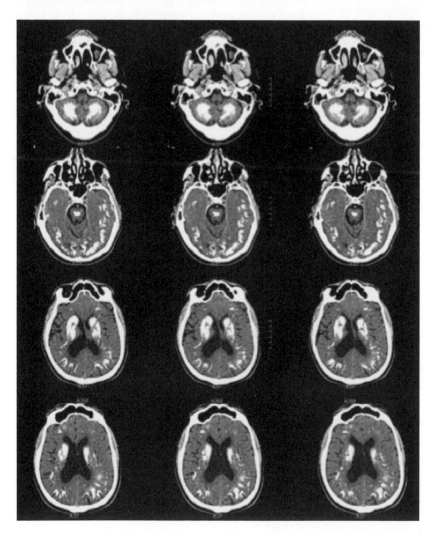

Figure 9.2 CT scan showing widespread calcifications, especially within the basal ganglia and cerebellum.

Table 9.1 Known genes and loci associated with primary familial brain calcification

Former locus denomination*	Gene	Chromosomal area	Inheritance
IBGC1 / IBGC3	SLC20A2	8p11	AD
IBGC2	unknown	2q37	–
IBGC4	PDGFRB	5q32	AD
IBGC5	PDGFB	22q12	AD
IBGC6	XPR1	1q25	AD

* The acronym IBGC (Idiopathic basal ganglia calcification) has been replaced by PFBC as it does not account for the fact that imaging abnormalities almost always extend beyond the basal ganglia.

As far as PFBC syndromes are concerned, both familial and non-familial cases have been reported, predominantly with autosomal-dominant fashion. The clinical presentation of PFBC is wide: symptoms begin in adulthood, usually in the fourth decade, and include movement disorders (mainly dystonia, ataxia, and parkinsonism), and psychiatric and cognitive problems including difficulty concentrating, memory loss, and changes in personality. Frequently, patients can have headache or migraine, while rarely they can present with seizures. The severity of PFBC also varies among affected individuals, with some people (up to 50 per cent) being completely asymptomatic.

Four genes, all inherited in a dominant fashion, have been found so far to cause PFBC (Table 9.1). On the contrary, a number of cases with PFBC, as our patient, do not have a family history or mutations in such genes, hence suggesting genetic heterogeneity for this condition. Mutations in the SLC20A2 gene have been estimated to cause nearly half of all cases of (familial) PBGC. The SLC20A2 gene encodes protein called sodium-dependent phosphate transporter 2, which plays a major role in regulating phosphate levels within the body. As a result, SLC20A2 mutations cause raised phosphate levels that combines with calcium and forms deposits. A small percentage of cases are instead caused by mutations in the PDGFRB gene. The mechanisms thereby PDGFRB mutations cause PFBC are unclear. Interestingly, mutations in the PDGF-B gene have been also associated with PFBC. PDGF-B encodes the platelet-derived growth factor beta polypeptide, which is the main ligand of PDGFRB, suggesting that

this pathway is crucial for brain calcium homeostasis. It is proposed that mutation in either of these two genes alters pericite and brain-blood barrier permeability to phosphate, thus leading to deposits of calcium phosphate. XPR1 gene encodes a protein that mediates phosphate export across the membrane. Deficits of this protein are expected to increase the concentration of the intracellular phosphate.

Given the paucity of patients with mutation of known genes for PFBC reported so far, it is hard to speculate on the possible link between severity and location of calcifications and clinical or genetic characteristics. Similarly, prognosis is uncertain, raising particular challenges for the counseling of mutation carriers.

Suggested Readings

Tadic V, Westenberger A, Domingo A, Alvarez-Fischer D, Klein C, Kasten M. Primary familial brain calcification with known gene mutations: a systematic review and challenges of phenotypic characterization. *JAMA Neurol*. 2015 Feb. 16. doi: 10.1001/jamaneurol.2014.3889.

Taglia I, Mignarri A, Olgiati S, et al. Primary familial brain calcification: genetic analysis and clinical spectrum. *Mov Disord*. 2014;29:1691–5.

 Video 9.1

Speech stuttering and freezing of gait, mainly on turning.

Case

10

A (Familial) PSP Look-Alike: Perry Syndrome

Roberto Erro, Maria Stamelou, and Kailash P. Bhatia

Clinical History

This 60-year-old woman presented to our department for a 4-year history of shaking of her hands. She is from a sibship of eight, of whom two older brothers were reported to have tremor. Moreover, her mother died around the age of 70 following a decade or more of a tremulous illness.

When she first started having tremor, a general practitioner diagnosed PD and put her on levodopa (300 md/day), to which she beneficially responded. However, she significantly progressed over the years and started complaining about walking difficulties and poor balance, but she had no actual falls. Her husband further reported that she had become extremely apathetic and had withdrawn from familial activities and social interactions.

Examination

On examination (Video 10.1), she was found to have a hypomimic face, with frontalis overactivity, and a staring expression. She had decreased upgaze with broken vertical saccades compared to horizontal saccades. She was hypokinetic in her upper limbs without evident asymmetry, whereas her gait was within normal limits for her age, beyond absent arm-swinging. Her pull-test was negative. Furthermore, she had brisk reflexes throughout along with a positive left palmomental reflex and an up-going plantar on the right side. There was a supinator catch indicating spastic tone rather than rigidity in the arms. No tremor was visible and the remaining examination was normal, besides a clear difficulty in engaging with the patient.

General Remarks

Although some features in this case might be reminiscent of PSP-P (cf. Case 6), including the initial presentation with tremor and the positive response to levodopa along with the development of an abnormal ocular motility, there were some atypical aspects one would not expect in a patient with classic PSP. First, there was a positive family history with an autosomal dominant pattern of inheritance. Second, certain findings on examination were pointing to a pyramidal involvement, which is not classically seen in PSP. The differential diagnosis in cases like this therefore includes rare genetic disorders of the FTD-MND spectrum.

Investigations and Diagnosis

A brain MRI proved to be normal, while she had an abnormal DaT-Scan. Central motor conduction studies disclosed abnormal findings, confirming the involvement of the pyramidal system. A genetic panel for the FTD-MND spectrum was hence requested and she was found to carry the heterozygous mutation c.A220G in the *Dynactin 1* (*DCTN1*) gene, leading to the diagnosis of Perry syndrome.

Special Remarks

Perry syndrome is a progressive neurodegenerative disease, underpinned pathologically by TDP-43 inclusions, due to mutations in the *DCTN1* gene. The penetrance of the disorder is estimated to be about 50 per cent. Clinically, it is characterized by four major features: parkinsonism, psychiatric changes, weight loss, and abnormally slow breathing (hypoventilation). Parkinsonism and psychiatric changes (e.g. athymhormia, apathy, hallucinations) are usually the earliest features of Perry syndrome, occurring between age 30 and 60. Parkinsonian features can respond to levodopa and there have been reports of development of motor fluctuations and dyskinesias. The most frequent psychiatric changes that occur in people with Perry syndrome include depression, a general loss of interest and enthusiasm (apathy), withdrawal from friends and family, and suicidal thoughts (which might be one cause of death in these patients).

Characteristically, many affected individuals also experience significant, unexplained weight loss and respiratory difficulties, most often occurring at night and causing them to wake up frequently. As the disease progresses, hypoventilation can result in respiratory failure and this is in fact the most common cause whereby affected individuals ultimately die, approximately 5 or 6 years after signs first have appeared.

Extreme apathy, weight loss, and hypoventilation are important clues to suspect Perry syndrome, along with a dominant family history, but it is essential to remark that the family history could be negative for a movement disorder as *DCTN1* mutations have also been reported to produce MDN alone, FTD alone, or a combination of phenotypes.

Suggested Readings

Perry TL, Wright JM, Berry K, Hansen S, Perry TL Jr. Dominantly inherited apathy, central hypoventilation, and Parkinson's syndrome: clinical, biochemical, and neuropathologic studies of 2 new cases. *Neurology*. 1990;40:1882–7.

Stamelou M, Quinn NP, Bhatia KP. 'Atypical' parkinsonism: new genetic conditions presenting with features of progressive supranuclear palsy, corticobasal degeneration, or multiple system atrophy. *Mov Disord*. 2013;28(9):1184–99.

Wider C, Dachsel JC, Farrer MJ, Dickson DW, Tsuboi Y, Wszolek ZK. Elucidating the genetics and pathology of Perry syndrome. *J Neurol Sci*. 2010;289:149–54.

 Video 10.1

There is frontalis overcativity and she has a staring expression. Ocular movements are very restricted upwards, but only partially correctable with the eye-doll manoeuvre. There is no clear appendicular bradykinesia.

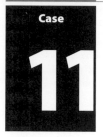

Parkinsonian Syndrome and Sunflower Cataracts: Wilson's Disease

Roberto Erro and Kailash P. Bhatia

Clinical History

This 30-year-old right-handed man, with no family history, developed difficulty walking and playing tennis since past 2 years. Symptoms were progressive and he slowed down remarkably during this period of time. In the last year, he also developed a tremor in his right hand. He felt he had lost the feel for his tennis shots with his right arm with further deterioration of the above symptoms. His speech also became affected.

Examination

On examination (Video 11.1), it was found that he had a hypomimic face, but ocular movements and cranial nerves were normal. He had mild dysarthria. There was an intermittent rest tremor and a postural tremor of his right arm. He had bilateral akinetic-rigid parkinsonism, with bradykinesia on tapping tasks. Moreover, he had micrographia. There was clear dystonic posturing of his neck. His gait was unsteady, and his postural reflexes mildly affected. The remaining neurological examination was normal.

General Remarks

The dominant feature in this case was undoubtedly that of a parkinsonian syndrome. However, there were also some red-flags, including dystonia, imbalance, and a mildly dysarthric speech, possibly denoting a cerebellar involvement. The syndromic association is most helpful to lead the diagnostic work-up in cases like this one. In fact, most of the monogenic forms of early onset parkinsonism (cf. Table 3.1) typically do not have cerebellar features. Hence, one would first consider those conditions where parkinsonism associates with a cerebellar involvement. Such a differential diagnosis is relatively short and includes WD, some forms of SCAs, PLAN, and MSA-C. However, the latter possibility is most unlikely given the age at onset in our patient. Among the most common types of SCAs, SCA2, SCA3 (Machado–Joseph disease), SCA8, and SCA17 can

present with parkinsonism. Even the 'purest' of the SCAs, namely SCA6, has been rarely reported to feature parkinsonism. Nevertheless, one would have expected a higher cerebellar burden (and a possible family history) in any of these conditions. Moreover, although any of these SCAs can present in the late twenties, this is not usually the rule. A cerebellar syndrome related to PLAN is a reasonable possibility, given that cerebellar features are frequently described in this disorder. However, one should first rule out WD, which (1) is a treatable disorder, and (2) is more prevalent, despite being a relatively rare disorder.

Investigations and Diagnosis

Serum ceruloplasmin was low (0.03 g/L) and 24-h urine copper was raised. A slit-lamp examination revealed the presence of Kayser–Fleischer rings bilaterally (cf. Figure 45.1). Moreover, there was evidence of early 'sunflower cataracts', suggestive of copper deposition in the lens capsule. A brain MRI showed T2-weighted hyperintense signal in the putamen and external pallidus, bilaterally (Figure 11.1B). Furthermore, the 'face of the giant panda' (which is pathognomonic of WD) in the midbrain with high signal in tegmentum and normal red nuclei was present (Figure 11.1A). A DaT-Scan was normal. He was confirmed compound heterozygous for the c.1336G>C mutation in exon 3 and the c.2866-13G>C mutation in exon 13 of the *ATP7B* gene, thus confirming a diagnosis of WD.

Special Remarks

WD is an autosomal recessive condition characterized by copper accumulation in several tissues and organs, due to mutations in the *ATP7B* gene, which encodes a copper-transporting P-type ATPase. The exact prevalence of WD is not clear. One genetic study has suggested that the prevalence of homozygous carriers can be as high as 1 in 7,000 individuals, which is substantially higher than the number of clinically diagnosed

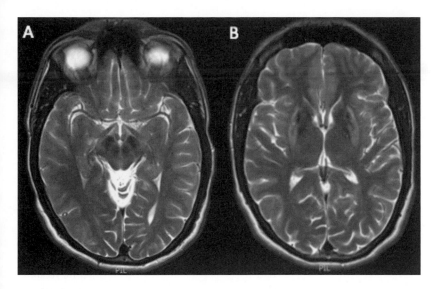

Figure 11.1 T2 weighted MRI imaging showing: (A) the 'face of the giant panda' sign in the midbrain with high signal in tegmentum and normal red nuclei; and (B) hyperintense signal in the putamen and external pallidus, bilaterally.

patients, hence raising the possibility that quite a number of WD cases are missed.

The main sites of copper accumulation are the liver and the brain, and consequently liver disease and neuropsychiatric symptoms are the main features of WD. Patients who manifest liver problems tend to come to medical attention earlier, generally as children or teenagers. Conversely, neurological symptoms typically begin in the second or third decade of life, with only 4 per cent or less becoming symptomatic after 40 years of age. However, late onset WD is well documented (seldom the onset can also be above the age of 70) and, hence, the diagnosis of WD should never be neglected because a patient is too old.

Clinically, patients with WD can be very heterogeneous, and the frequency of distinct neurological features varies widely in different case series. Classical features of WD include wing-beating tremor or the combination of dysarthria with slow tongue movements and orofacial dystonia or dyskinesias, including the 'risus sardonicus', a term describing involuntary grimacing with the mouth open and the upper lip contracted. In general, the presence of three more common neurological phenotypes have been suggested, namely, dystonic, ataxic, and parkinsonian or a combination of these, with further features including pyramidal signs, seizures, and psychiatric issues. Obviously, patients may have additional systemic signs and/or symptoms due to liver involvement, such as tiredness and increased bleeding tendency.

WD is relentlessly progressive and without treatment patients die from progressive liver failure or severe neurological disability. The two main therapeutic approaches are decoppering and liver transplant, which is performed in cases of rapidly progressive liver failure. Ideally, treatment should have two phases: an initial, acute de-coppering therapy and a subsequent maintenance therapy. Currently, penicillamine and trientine (triethylenetetramine) are the two oral copper chelators available for treatment of WD. Although there are no systematic head-to-head comparisons between these two drugs, trientine may have some advantage over penicillamine in being less immunogenic, but both drugs are safe and effective and may be used lifelong in patients with WD. In addition, zinc may be used in presymptomatic patients and during the maintenance phase of treatment of symptomatic patients, but it is not adequate as monotherapy in the initial intensive decoppering phase of treatment in symptomatic patients, since it is not a copper-chelator but inhibits intestinal copper absorption, thus having a negligible potential to mobilize copper from tissues that are already overloaded. The combination of zinc with either penicillamine or trientine presents significant dosing issues since both the latter can potentially chelate zinc, and should therefore be avoided.

Paradoxical worsening of the neurological symptoms is reported in up to 20 per cent of patients after initiation of chelation therapy with either copper chelators. The mechanism of this neurological deterioration is not fully understood, but it should not justify stopping the medications, since non-adherence or discontinuation of medical therapy is associated with the risk of intractable hepatic decompensation.

Suggested Readings

Aggarwal A, Bhatt M. The pragmatic treatment of Wilson's disease. *Mov Disord Clin Pract*. 2014;1(1):14–23.

Compston A. Progressive lenticular degeneration: a familial nervous disease associated with cirrhosis of the liver, by SA Kinnier Wilson, (From the National Hospital, and the Laboratory of the National Hospital, Queen Square, London). *Brain*. 1912:34;295–509. *Brain*. 2009;132:1997–2001.

Lorincz MT. Recognition and treatment of neurologic Wilson's disease. *Semin Neurol*. 2012;32(5):538–43.

 Video 11.1

This patient has reduced blink rate and a retrocollis. On finger tapping there is bradykinesia (left>right). He walks with a stooped posture and short steps. Arm swing is reduced and arms are held in a flexed position.

Case

12

Classic PD-Like Rest Tremor in FTDP-17 Due to a *MAPT* Mutation

Roberto Erro, Stephanie T. Hirschbichler, and Kailash P. Bhatia

Clinical History

A 56-year-old, right-handed lady of Latin American origin with a positive family history for dementia (her mother had been diagnosed with AD late in life), experienced a 7-month history of rest tremor of her right hand and general slowness and had therefore been put on pergolide, 3 mg per day, reporting a subjective good response. Accordingly, she was diagnosed with PD by a general neurologist. Her family members, however, complained shortly after about her having become forgetful and sleepy, although she herself was not aware of any cognitive and behavioural issues. She was hence referred to us for a second opinion. There were no reports of hallucinations, cognitive and/or motor fluctuations, or night-time sleep problems.

Examination

There was an asymmetric parkinsonian syndrome featuring rest tremor of the right hand, along with an asymmetric bilateral tremor (right>left) and dystonic posturing of the hands on posture. There was relatively mild bradykinesia and rigidity of the right upper and lower limb. In addition, there was some difficulty with coping gestures with her left hand (see Video 12.1) in the absence of ideomotor apraxia. The remaining neurological examination, including eye movements, was unremarkable. Bedside cognitive examination was unremarkable although she appeared 'disinhibited', suggesting some frontal involvement.

General Remarks

Mood dysfunction and apathy are relatively common in PD, even in the earliest stage. However, they usually do not overshadow motor symptoms and, in fact, patients most commonly seek medical advice when the latter appear. Cognitive impairment can also be seen in early PD patients, but troublesome memory issues and/or frank dementia are again seen only in the advanced stages of the disease. Indeed, significant early

cognitive dysfunctions are one of the exclusion benchmarks, according to the UK Brain Bank criteria for PD. Thus, the presence of early cognitive impairment in our patient (and the possible autosomal dominant family history for dementia) would suggest an alternative diagnosis. Several conditions, including the monogenic forms of parkinsonism, can give rise to such a phenotype (cf. Case 4). However, given the diagnosis of AD in her mother, such disorders in which dementia is the core feature and parkinsonism may occur (i.e. FTD, which in some cases can be misdiagnosed with AD), should be considered first, especially if a particular pattern of cortical atrophy on imaging is observed.

Investigations and Diagnosis

A brain MRI turned out to be normal (no significant atrophy) and a DaT-Scan confirmed presynaptic nigro-striatal degeneration. A formal neuropsychometry disclosed marked cognitive decline compared to premorbid estimates (verbal IQ of 73, performance IQ of 59) and significant impairment of both executive functions and visuo-spatial processing. Given the possible autosomal dominant family history for dementia and the early development of cognitive and behavioural dysfunction in our patient, further genetic testing for *PSEN1* and *PSEN2* (i.e. presenilin1 and 2), and *MAPT* was pursued and she was found positive for the previously described c.1216C>T *MAPT* mutation (p.r406w), thus leading to a definite diagnosis of FTDP-17 associated with a *MAPT* mutation.

Special Remarks

In the early 1990s, an international consensus conference was held to define the association of parkinsonism with FTD, and the term FTDP-17 was introduced. Subsequently, mutations in two different genes on chromosome 17, namely *MAPT* encoding the microtubule-associated protein tau and *PGRN* encoding progranulin, have been associated with FTDP-17,

Table 12.1 Overview of the Genes Associated with Parkinsonism in FTD

	MAPT	PRGN	C9ORF72	CHMP2B	VCP	TARDBP	FUS
Localization	17q21.32	17q.21.31	9p21.2	3p11.2	9p13.3	1p36.22	16p11.2
Inheritance	Autosomal dominant	Autosomal dominant	Autosomal dominant	Autosomal dominant	Autosomal dominant	Autosomal dominant	Autosomal dominant
Penetrance	Almost 100%	90% by age 70 years	NE (probably high)	NE	Incomplete	NE	NE
Estimated frequency in FTD	Up to 50%	3–26%	14–48%	<1%	<1%	<1%	<1%
Average age at onset (range)	49 years (25–76)	59 years (44–83)	55 years (33–75)	58 years (46–71)	55 years (37–79)	54 years (35–74)	43 years (30–60)
Presence of parkinsonism	Frequent	Relatively common	Relatively common	Relatively common	Rare	Relatively common	Rare
Prominent neuropathology	Tau	TDP-43 (transactive DNA-binding protein)	TDP-43/ Ubiquitin	Ubiquitin	TDP-43	TDP-43	FUS (fused in sarcome protein)

Source: Adapted from Siuda J, Fujioka S, Wszolek ZK. Parkinsonian syndrome in familial frontotemporal dementia. *Parkinsonism Relat. Disord.* 2014;20(9):957–64.

despite the fact that other genes not located on chromosome 17 (Table 12.1) can produce a similar phenotype. *MAPT* mutations account for the large majority of cases of FTD and associated parkinsonism. In this context, parkinsonian features are usually symmetrical and often characterized by severe bradykinesia, rigidity, and postural instability, with no rest tremor. Instead, symmetrical postural/action tremor might be seldom observed. Furthermore, atypical features including oculomotor abnormalities and supranuclear upgaze palsy, bulbar symptoms, and/or corticospinal tract involvement can be observed. Parkinsonism often occurs early in the disease and might respond to levodopa treatment, although the response is usually not sustained. Therefore, the parkinsonism observed in FTDP-17 due to *MAPT* mutations does not classically feature rest tremor and does not resemble PD. The presence of classical rest tremor is hence quite unusual in FTDP-17 and in fact our patient has been initially misdiagnosed with PD. Recognition of this disorder is important for genetic counselling and to the treatment, especially because dopaminergic drugs can cause or exacerbate psychiatric symptoms in these patients,

and thus an adequate balance of benefits with potential risks needs to be achieved.

Suggested Readings

Baizabal-Carvallo JF, Jankovic J. Parkinsonism, movement disorders and genetics in frontotemporal dementia. *Nat. Rev. Neurol.* 2016;12:175-85.

Galimberti D, Scarpini E. Clinical phenotypes and genetic biomarkers of FTLD. *J Neural Transm.* 2012;119(7):851–60.

Siuda J, Fujioka S, Wszolek ZK. Parkinsonian syndrome in familial frontotemporal dementia. *Parkinsonism Relat. Disord.* 2014;20(9):957–64.

 Video 12.1

There is an irregular rest tremor of the right hand, along with an asymmetric bilateral tremor (right>left) and dystonic posturing of the hands on posture. Moreover, there is a mild bradykinesia of the right hand. There is some difficulty with copying gestures, particularly with her left hand.

Case

13

PSP Look-Alike due to CADASIL

Roberto Erro and Paolo Barone

Clinical History

This 76-year-old man developed slowness of gait, apathy, depression, and minor memory issues 4 years earlier. His symptoms were slowly progressive and he sought medical advice only 3 years into his disease, when he further started having unexplained falls. He was admitted into another hospital, where a diagnosis of possible PSP (cf. Case 5) was made, also owing to the evidence of supranuclear upgaze palsy on examination and ineffective L-dopa therapy. Four years after onset, he was referred to us for a second opinion. Collateral history was taken from caregivers, who besides the aforementioned symptoms and signs, reported mild dysphagia and very occasional urinary incontinence. Worth of note, there was positive family history for cerebrovascular accidents: his father had died of a stroke at 56 years and his sister had recurrent strokes in her forties.

Examination

On examination (Video 13.1), he had a hypomimic face with a staring expression. There was a clear upgaze supranuclear palsy with slow saccades in the vertical plane. He further had a severe parkinsonism featuring severe bradykinesia, marked rigidity (axial > appendicular), and positive pull test. Unaided walking was impossible. He had brisk reflexes, and palmomental and glabellar tap reflexes were present, along with perseverative responses during the applause test. The remaining neurological examination was normal.

General Remarks

Although the overall phenotype of this patient bears resemblance with that of PSP (cf. Case 5), there were some unusual features that do not entirely fit in with the 'classic' description of this disorder. Indeed, age at onset in this case was slightly above that observed in PSP, where patients usually start having symptoms during their sixth decade. This observation on its own should prompt pursuing an extensive diagnostic work-up to exclude different disorders, which might masquerade as PSP. NPH can in fact present with a PSP-like phenotype and should be considered when gait and balance disturbances, urinary incontinence, and cognitive decline (i.e. the classical clinical triad of NPH) occur. However, the family history of cerebrovascular disease at a relatively young onset cannot be ignored and raises the possibility of a genetically transmitted leukoencephalopathy, including CADASIL, HDLS (cf. Case 15), and Alexander disease, that can rarely present with a PSP-like syndrome.

Investigations and Diagnosis

Extensive laboratory study revealed normal findings. Brain MRI showed significant basal ganglia lesions and white matter hyperintensities, including periventricular regions and both frontal and temporal subcortical areas, along with moderate widespread atrophy and ventricular enlargement (Figure 13.1). A DaT-Scan was performed which yielded normal results. Given the imaging results along with the family history for early cerebrovascular disease, genetic screening of the NOTCH3 gene was performed and this patient was found to carry a heterozygous NOTCH3 mutation (c.C307T), leading to the diagnosis of CADASIL.

Special Remarks

CADASIL is an autosomal dominant cerebral small-vessel disease due to mutations in the NOTCH3 gene, which most commonly appears in early/middle adulthood with frequent headache of migraine pattern, focal deficits secondary to recurrent strokes, and, in later stages, progressive neuropsychiatric disorders leading to a frank dementia. However, late onset cases (after age 60 years) with atypical phenotypes have been reported. In fact, another CADASIL case has been reported with a PSP-like syndrome and it has been unveiled that parkinsonism may be a common but unrecognized manifestation of CADASIL.

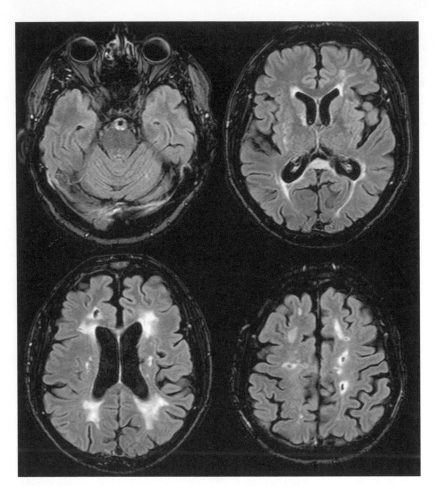

Figure 13.1 Axial fluid-attenuated inversion recovery images showing areas of abnormal signal within the basal ganglia and white matter hyperintensities of periventricular regions and both frontal and temporal subcortical areas.

More generally, gait problems, urinary incontinence, and pseudobulbar symptoms and signs seem to be also extremely frequent in this condition. Therefore, mutations in the *NOTCH3* gene should be considered in all cases of parkinsonism with: (1) imaging consistent with a leukoencephalopathy; and (2) family history for cerebrovascular disease. In this context, it is important to remark that up to one-third of CADASIL cases apparently have a negative family history. This is likely owing to a restricted search only for classic cases in the family (e.g. with migraine and early onset strokes) and not for uncommon presentations of CADASIL, including epileptic syndromes, complex and acute encephalopathies, or, as in this case, 'atypical' parkinsonism.

Suggested Readings

Moccia M, Mosca L, Erro R, et al. Hypomorphic NOTCH3 mutation in an Italian family with CADASIL features. *Neurobiol Aging.* 2015;36(1):547.e5–11.

Ragno M, Berbellini A, Cacchiò G, et al. Parkinsonism is a late, not rare, feature of CADASIL. *Stroke.* 2013;44(4):1147–9.

Stamelou M, Quinn NP, Bhatia KP. 'Atypical' atypical parkinsonism: new genetic conditions presenting with features of progressive supranuclear palsy, corticobasal degeneration, or multiple system atrophy. *Mov Disord.* 2013;28(9):1184–99.

 Video 13.1

There is frontalis overactivity and the patient has a staring expression. Ocular smooth pursuits are restricted on the vertical plane. Saccades are slow and hypometric on the vertical plane as compared to the horizontal one. There is bradykinesia, especially on the left and frontal release signs. Gait is impossible without support, also owing to severe imbalance.

Very Early Onset Parkinsonism: Juvenile HD

Roberto Erro and Kailash P. Bhatia

Clinical History

A 62-year-old woman developed stiffness in her movements by the age of 6 years. Her adoptive parents noted paucity and slowness of her movements, following a viral infection where she had been encephalopatic. Despite her complete recovery from the infection, symptoms were progressive over the years. Nevertheless, activities of daily living were well maintained until her early adulthood. Over time, she consulted a number of neurologists, but only a working diagnosis of early onset Parkinsonism, possibly related to the viral infection, was made. A trial of levodopa was proven unsuccessful and she did not consult any neurologists for a number of years. She was, however, under the care of a psychiatrist for the development of a severe apathetic syndrome with additional depression and memory complaints. A further progression of her symptoms occurred, with the development of swallowing difficulties and with her having become wheelchair bound and totally dependent for her daily life activities. She therefore came to see us. No additional information was available as to her biological family.

Examination

On examination (see Video 14.1), it was found that saccades were slow with increased latency. She was found to be severely hypomimic, with a staring expression, and hypophonic. She had a laterocollis to the right. There was severe bradykinesia in both arms, while she could not perform foot tapping at all. There was both truncal and appendicular rigidity. She was wheelchair bound, and unaided walking was impossible. The remaining neurological examination was normal.

General Remarks

Although the suspicion of post-encephalitic parkinsonism, despite being extremely rare, would have been reasonable in this case, there were a number of missing characteristics that would argue against such

a diagnosis. Post-encephalitic parkinsonism typically has at least three of the following: signs of basal ganglia involvement; ophthalmoplegia; oculogyric crises; obsessive-compulsive behavior; akinetic mutism; central respiratory irregularities; and somnolence or sleep inversion, occurring after an acute or subacute encephalitic illness. None of these, apart from the parkinsonism, was present in our patient, making such a diagnosis very unlikely.

On the contrary, the combination of an akinetic-rigid syndrome, with cognitive and psychiatric features at this age has a wide differential diagnosis. Two conditions that are important in this context are WD and the Westphal variant of HD. However, neurological WD does not occur below age 7. Other rare genetic causes of parkinsonism (cf. Table 3.1) may present with a similar phenotype. Furthermore, certain conditions, including dopamine transporter deficiency, deficits in the dopamine synthesis pathway or NBIA, can present with this phenotype, but they usually, if not invariably, have additional features such as oculogyric crises, hypothonia, delayed milestones, and pyramidal signs.

Investigations and Diagnosis

A brain MRI revealed generalized cortical atrophy and a marked volume loss in the caudate nucleus bilaterally (Figure 14.1), which was suggestive of HD. A genetic testing was pursued and she was found to have a pathological expansion (85 CAG triplets) in the IT15 gene, thus confirming the diagnosis of HD.

Special Remarks

The Westphal variant of HD is a distinct clinical entity, which is characterized by a rigid-akinetic syndrome and usually associated with a juvenile onset of the disease. Although the typical age of onset of HD is in the fourth decade of life (cf. Case 34), between 5 and 10 per cent of cases have a onset before the age of 20 years, with symptoms developing before the age of

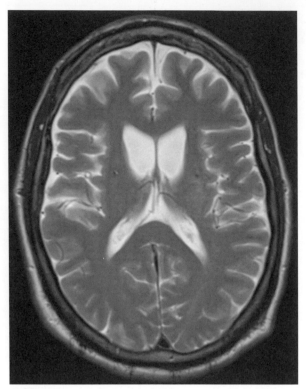

Figure 14.1 Axial MR image showing marked caudate volume loss and frontal cortical atrophy.

5 years being rather exceptional. There is a significant correlation between the number of CAG repeats, and the age at onset of disease and repeat number over 60 is invariably associated with onset before 20 years of age, but substantial variability remains. It is clear that in the majority of such cases, the transmission is from the paternal side due to meiotic instability and expansion of the CAG repeat. Moreover, parkinsonian paternal cases have a significantly lower age at onset, as well as a shorter duration of disease than choreatic paternal cases, whereas no such relationship exists between parkinsonian maternal and choreatic maternal cases.

The clinical features of the Westphal variant sensibly differ from those of the common adult onset form of HD. In fact, children with HD often show a preponderance of rigidity, dystonia, bradykinesia, learning disabilities, seizures, and myoclonus, whereas choreic movements can be completely absent. Furthermore, there is also a more rapid disease progression than in the adult onset form.

An overview on the HD is provided in Case 34, and we wish to remark that HD should be considered in the differential diagnosis of neurodegenerative parkinsonism in children, even in the absence of a positive family history.

Suggested Readings

Nance MA, Myers RH. Juvenile onset Huntington's disease- clinical and research perspectives. *Ment Retard Dev Disabil Res Rev.* 2001;7:153–7.

Rasmussen A, Marcias R, Yescas P, Ochoa A, Davila G, Alonso E. Huntington disease in children. Genotype-phenotype correlation. *Neuropediatrics.* 2000;31:190–4.

 Video 14.1

This patient is wheelchair bound. She has hypomimia and a laterocollis to the right. There is a tremor in her right arm on posture and there is marked hypokinesia.

Case

15

Parkinsonism Due to *CSF1R* Mutation

David S Lynch, Zane Jaunmuktane, and Henry Houlden

Clinical History

A 47-year-old man with no family history for any neurological disorders presented with a 2-year history of personality change and depression. He had used intravenous drugs sporadically since his twenties and had chronic Hepatitis C as a result. His drug use had accelerated prior to his presentation. He made reckless financial decisions and became violent at home. Within 6 months of this presentation, he developed upper limb apraxia and went on to develop a clear parkinsonian gait with prominent freezing and frequent falls. His condition deteriorated over time and was further complicated by cognitive problems.

Examination

On examination, upper limb apraxia and a parkinsonian gait with prominent freezing and frequent falls were found. Eye movements were impaired with slow saccades, visual impersistence, and supranuclear gaze palsy. There was severe axial and appendicular rigidity, with rest tremor and stimulus sensitive myoclonus in his left upper limb. Speech was dysarthric but there were no other bulbar or pyramidal features.

General Remarks

The main phenotype in this case could have raised the suspicion of an atypical parkinsonism, particularly PSP and/or CBS (cf. Cases 5, 6, and 7); however, the age at onset – 45 years – would be unusual for either. The differential diagnosis for an atypical parkinsonism complicated by dementia is broad and mainly includes neurometabolic and genetic causes of parkinsonism. Also, given the history of intravenous drug use, one should also consider the possibility of an infectious or immune-mediated disorder. The diagnostic work-up in cases like this should be accordingly broad and some of the investigations, particularly the imaging (MRI and DaT-Scan), are fundamental since they allow narrowing the differential diagnosis.

Investigations and Diagnosis

An extensive metabolic and autoimmune screen was normal, including HIV serology, VDRL, cryoglobulins, heavy metals, antineuronal and antibasal ganglia antibodies and CSF PCR for JC Virus and Whipple's disease. A brain MRI demonstrated extensive symmetrical T2 high signal in the cerebral white matter involving the frontal, parietal, and posterior temporal lobes (Figure 15.1), with the lateral and third ventricles being enlarged due to cerebral volume loss. A DaT-Scan was normal while a brain FDG-PET scan of the brain demonstrated reduced tracer uptake in the frontal and right parietal lobes (Figure 15.2). Genetic studies for HD, DRPLA, and CADASIL were negative. A brain biopsy was performed, demonstrating myelin pallor and reduced axon density towards deep white matter, where frequent axonal spheroids and scattered pigmented microglial cells were seen (Figure 15.3). Sequencing of the *CSF1R* gene was hence pursued, revealing a heterozygous p.A763P mutation in exon 19 and leading to the diagnosis of HDLS.

Special Remarks

HDLS is an autosomal dominant disorder due to *CSF1R* mutations, with symptomatic onset in midlife and death within a few years after symptom onset. CSF1R is a receptor expressed on microglia promoting cell survival, proliferation, and differentiation. HDLS has joined a growing list of 'microgliopathies', or primary disorders of microglia, often associated with early cognitive decline. In fact, patients carrying *CSF1R* mutations most frequently present with cognitive decline and depression, but additional features are common and may include parkinsonism in up to 45 per cent of cases as well as pyramidal signs, seizures, and ataxia. In fact, a large series has shown that a subset of HDLS patients fulfils clinical criteria for either PSP or CBS. Furthermore, in some patients parkinsonism can be the initial symptom and can dominate the clinical picture

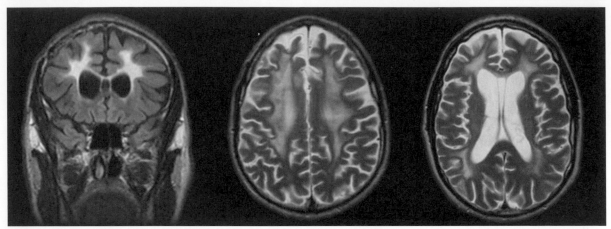

Figure 15.1 MRI imaging illustrating confluent, symmetrical high signal in the deep white matter of the frontal, parietal, and posterior temporal lobe.

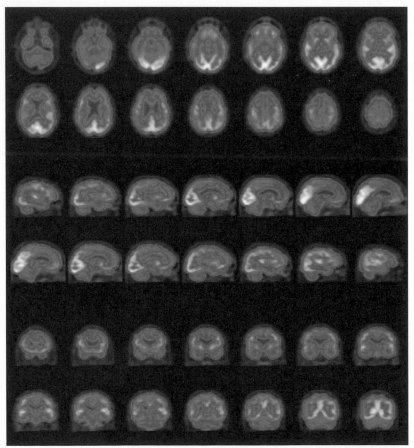

Figure 15.2 FDG-PET scan of the brain demonstrating reduced tracer uptake in the frontal and right parietal lobe. A black and white version of this figure will appear in some formats. For the colour version, please refer to the plate section.

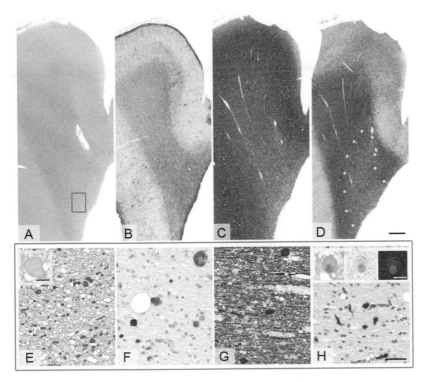

Figure 15.3 Full thickness brain biopsy. The Hematoxylin and Eosin (H&E) stain (A), immunostaining for glial fibrillary acid protein (B), axons (neurofilament cocktail), (C) and myelin (Luxol fast blue/cresyl violet) (D) shows a mild pallor of the myelin and reduction of axon density towards the deep white matter (separated by a yellow dotted line in D) where frequent axonal spheroids are seen (inset in E). The axonal spheroids label with antibodies for neurofilaments (E), amyloid precursor protein (F), and ubiquitin (G). Increased numbers of CD68 positive microglial cells are present in the deeper white matter (H), which show yellow–light brown cytoplasm on H&E and negative control sections and appear blue when viewed as a negative colour inversion image (insets in H). *(Scale bar: 1mm in A–D, 5µm in E–H, 10µm insets in E and H.)* A black and white version of this figure will appear in some formats. For the colour version, please refer to the plate section.

during the progression of the disease. In approximately 25 per cent of patients there is no family history and therefore such a disorder should be considered in sporadic cases with a compatible MRI scan (or with evidence of or axonal spheroids on brain biopsy).

MRI features are of symmetric, confluent white matter hyperintensities on T2 weighted imaging with thinning of the corpus callosum. Frequently there is DWI positivity, indicating restricted diffusion. This finding can, however, wax and wane over serial imaging, often raising suspicion of CNS vasculitis. At autopsy, the pathology is mainly restricted to the white matter, where axonal and myelin loss, accumulation of axonal spheroids and pigmented microglia is observed. These morphological changes usually vary in severity between cases, subject to the stage of the disease, biopsy site, and regional predilection for pathology, which predominantly affects the frontal and parietal lobes.

Suggested Readings

Sundal C, Fujioka S, Van Gerpen JA, et al. Parkinsonian features in hereditary diffuse leukoencephalopathy with spheroids (HDLS) and CSF1R mutations. *Parkinsonism Relat Disord.* 2013;19:869–77.

Guerreiro R, Kara E, Le Ber I et al. Genetic analysis of inherited leukodystrophies: Genotype–phenotype correlations in the CSF1R gene. *JAMA Neurol.* 2013;70:875–82.

Sundal C, Van Gerpen JA, Nicholson AM et al. MRI characteristics and scoring in HDLS due to CSF1R gene mutations. *Neurology.* 2012;79:566–74.

Early Onset Generalized Dystonia: DYT1

Roberto Erro and Kailash P. Bhatia

Clinical History

This 41-year-old woman, with no family history for any neurological disorders, had first started having walking difficulties at the age of 10. At that time she became aware that her right leg would pull up and make her walk awkwardly. Shortly afterwards she also noticed that when trying to pick something with her right hand, she would twist it in an unusual way. Her left limbs were instead entirely fine. She sought medical care for her symptoms, which were described as hemi-dystonia by the consultant neurologist, and a brain MRI was hence performed to exclude structural lesions. This turned out to be entirely normal and a diagnosis of idiopathic dystonia was made. However, 2–3 years later, her neck also started to be affected, turning towards the right side. Moreover, she also developed a stammer, but her voice was otherwise unchanged and she had no swallowing difficulties. In the following years, symptoms progressed further and she found that, when sitting down, she had to put her left leg over the right one to prevent her trunk bending forward. She was put on trihexyphenydil and benzodiazepines with gradual improvement and was then lost at follow-up because for a number of years her symptoms remained stable and were minimally affecting her functioning.

At the age of 35, she decided to stop her medications and around 1–2 years later her symptoms worsened and became troublesome. She reported that, when standing and walking, she would not be able to control her legs and would fall, needing to lean on something. She further reported the development of a bilateral leg tremor.

Examination

On examination, it was found that she had a mobile torticollis to the right with left laterocollis. There was no evidence of orofacial dystonia. There was abnormal posturing of her hands and she has difficulties when finger tapping with her left hand. Abnormal dystonic posturing was present also in her lower limbs, with her feet being turned outwards (Video 16.1). Moreover, there was a postural leg tremor, which could at times be transmitted to the upper limbs. She walked with irregular strides, and a marked hyperlordosis was evident. The remaining neurological examination was unremarkable.

General Remarks

This woman presented with an isolated (formerly known as primary) dystonia which affected her trunk, neck, and both lower and upper limbs (hence being generalized) with onset early in life. Despite the symptoms not developing acutely, over a few months, the body distribution at onset (hemi-dystonia) correctly prompted the supervising neurologist to perform a brain MRI in order to exclude a structural lesion. The absence of any imaging abnormalities (and other neurological systems involvement) and further progression towards a generalized form (with a peculiar pattern from the lower limbs to the upper ones and trunk) are quite suggestive of the monogenic form of dystonia type 1 (DYT1). Less frequently, similar phenotypes can be associated with DYT6 due to mutations in the *THAP1* gene (Table 16.1). However, in a number of early onset generalized dystonia patients, genetic testing remains inconclusive.

Investigations

A repeated brain MRI was entirely normal. A genetic testing confirmed that she carried a three-base pair deletion c.907_909delGAG of *TOR1A*, thus confirming a diagnosis of DYT1. Unaffected family members were not available for testing.

Special Remarks

DYT1 typically presents in childhood or adolescence and only seldom in adulthood. Dystonic muscle contractions causing posturing of a hand, foot, or leg are

Table 16.1 DYT-Designated Loci

Locus (synonym)	Chromosome	Gene	Inheritance	Phenotype
DYT1	9q34	*TOR1A*	AD	Early onset, generalized
DYT2/DYT2-like	1p34.2–35	*HPCA*	AR	Early onset, generalized, most prominent in upper limbs and cranial-cervical regions
DYT3 (Lubag)	Xq13.1	*TAF1*	X-linked	Dystonia-parkinsonism
DYT4 (whispering dysphonia)	19p13.3	*TUBB4A*	AD	Generalized dystonia, whispering dysphonia, and 'hobby-horse' gait in some affected subjects
DYT5a (DRD, Segawa variant)	14q22.1-q22.2	*GCH1*	AD	Dystonia with concurrent or subsequent parkinsonism, diurnal worsening of symptoms, dramatic response to levodopa
DYT5b	11p15.5	*TH*	AR	Complicated DRD
DYT6	8p11.21	*THAP1*	AD	Adolescent onset, mostly segmental with upper limb and cervical involvement
DYT7	18pter-p11.32	Unknown	AD	Adult onset focal dystonia
DYT8	2q34	*MR-1*	AD	PNKD
DYT9 (identical to DYT18)	1p34-p22	*SLC2A1*	AD	PED with spasticity
DYT10	16p11.2-q12.1	*PRRT2*	AD	PKD
DYT11	7q21.3	*SGCE*	AD	Myoclonus-dystonia
DYT12	19q13	*ATP1A3*	AD	Rapid onset dystonia-parkinsonism
DYT13	1p36.32-p36.12.13	Unknown	AD	Early or late onset, focal or segmental dystonia
DYT14	14q13	Unknown	AD	Generalized dopa-responsive dystonia-parkinsonism with gait and postural disturbances
DYT15	18p11	Unknown	AD	Myoclonus-dystonia
DYT16	2q31.2	*PRKRA*	AR	Early onset dystonia-parkinsonism
DYT17	20p11.22-q13.12	*Unknown*	AR	Early onset generalized dystonia
DYT18	1p34-p22	*SLC2A1*	AD	PED (as part of GLUT-1 deficiency syndrome)
DYT19 (identical to DYT10)	16p11.2-q12.1	*PRRT2*	AD	PKD
DYT20 (identical to DYT8)	2q34	*MR-1*	AD	PNKD
DYT21	2q14.3-q21.3	Unknown	AD	Early to late onset, progression to generalized form with prominent cranial involvement
DYT23	9q34	*CIZ1*	AD	Late onset cervical dystonia
DYT24	11p14.2	*ANO3*	AD	Onset in early to middle adulthood; focal or segmental dystonia, with prominent cranial-cervical involvement and a tremulous component
DYT25	18p11.21	*GNAL*	AD	Adult onset cervical dystonia with possible progression to segmental dystonia
DYT26	22q12.3	*KCTD17*	AD	Myoclonus-dystonia
DYT27	2q37	*COL6A3*	AR	Early onset generalized dystonia

Abb.: AD: Autosomal dominant; AR: autosomal recessive; PNKD: paroxysmal non-kinesigenic dyskinesias; PKD: paroxysmal kinesigenic dyskinesias; PED: paroxysmal exercise-induced dyskinesias.

the most common presenting findings. Dystonia is usually first apparent with specific actions such as writing or walking but symptoms frequently, though not invariably, become evident with less specific actions and spread to other body regions over time. Selective or pronounced craniocervical involvement is said to be unusual. During the disease course, relatively long periods of remission have been reported. No other neurologic abnormalities are present, except for postural arm tremor. Disease severity varies considerably even within the same family, and segmental or focal forms such as isolated writer's cramp have been exceptionally described, especially if symptom onset is in adulthood.

DYT1 is the most common form of monogenic dystonia and it is inherited in an autosomal dominant fashion with reduced penetrance. The chance of developing clinical findings for *TOR1A* carriers have been estimated to range between 30 and 40 per cent. DYT1 is 5–10 times more common in subjects with Ashkenazi Jewish ancestry, despite the fact that it can occur in individuals of any ethnicity. The c.907_909delGAG deletion is the only definitive DYT1 disease-causing mutation identified so far and sequence analysis is hence unlikely to provide additional diagnostic information in an individual who does not have such a deletion. Other variants have been seldom identified in single affected individuals, but their true pathogenicity remains unknown. DYT1 genetic testing is recommended for symptomatic individuals with at least one of the following: isolated dystonia in any body region with onset before age 26 years; onset in a limb before the age of 30 years; and/or a family history of early onset dystonia.

Suggested Readings

Bressman SB, Sabatti C, Raymond D, et al. The DYT1 phenotype and guidelines for diagnostic testing. *Neurology*. 2000;54:1746–52.

Müller U. The monogenic primary dystonias. *Brain*. 2009;132:2005–25.

Valente EM, Warner TT, Jarman PR, et al. The role of DYT1 in primary torsion dystonia in Europe. *Brain*. 1998;121:2335–9.

 Video 16.1

This patient has a generalized dystonia affecting her trunk and lower limbs, with evident tremor. Her gait is dystonic and affected by the trunk involvement.

Early Onset Jerky Dystonia: An Uncommon Phenotype of DYT1

Roberto Erro and Kailash P. Bhatia

Clinical History

This 61-year-old woman first presented at the age of 10 years with difficulty in writing and necessity to change the hand to do so. Additional leg problems with posturing and minor difficulty in walking developed in her teens. In her early twenties, a head jerky tremor became evident and was her main complaint. Her tremor worsened over time and spread to the upper limbs, but she was able to carry on her day-to-day activities and succeeded in her job as journalist. She found that alcohol did not dramatically improve her tremor. As to her family history, she has a brother severely affected with early onset generalized dystonia, whereas her parents and her two daughters were deemed to be fine.

Examination

On examination (see Video 17.1), a jerky side-to-side tremor of her head was evident, with minimal abnormal posturing of her neck and trunk. Head movements were not particularly restricted. A jerky tremor, which changed in frequency and amplitude according to certain arm positions, was evident in her upper limbs. Moreover, excessive flexion of her right wrist was observed on posture. Lower limbs at rest were normal. Her walking was dystonic and further exacerbated her trunk dystonia. In addition, there were axial jerks. Writing with her right hand was almost impossible for the presence of wide jerky tremor. Left hand writing was also affected, but still possible. The remaining neurological examination was clear.

Investigations

Basic blood investigations and a brain MRI were normal. Given the positive family history and the early age at onset, genetic testing for DYT1 was pursued and she was found to carry the c.907_909del-GAG *TOR1A* mutation, thus leading to a diagnosis of DYT1.

Remarks

The very first symptom in this patient was a dystonic posturing on writing, which developed at the age of 10 years. Moreover, she has a positive family history, her brother being affected with early onset dystonia. Hence, according to current guidelines, she should have tested for DYT1 (cf. Case 16) and she was indeed found to carry a *TOR1A* mutation. However, her main complaint and most obvious finding on examination was a jerky tremor affecting her head and arms. Other DYT1 patients with similar phenotype have been described in the literature. Thus, a few DYT1 carriers have been reported on with predominant jerky tremor and/or myoclonus that overshadowed the dystonic features, so that myoclonus-dystonia (DYT11, cf. Table 16.1) was considered in the differential diagnosis. In our case, the phenotype, despite not being particularly prototypical for DYT1, was not typical for DYT11 either (cf. Case 52). In the latter, myoclonic jerks are brief, 'shock-like', usually in retrocollis, and a dramatic response to alcohol is seen.

As gene testing for the DYT1 mutation has become quite widespread in the previous years, it has emerged that the phenotype associated with DYT1 positivity can be rather broad. It is important to recognize atypical presentations of DYT1 as to genetic counseling and also because of the predictive value in terms of positive response to DBS.

Suggested Readings

Chinnery PF, Reading PJ, McCarthy EL, et al. Late onset axial jerky dystonia due to the DYT1 deletion. *Mov Disord*. 2002;17:196–8.

Edwards M, Wood N, Bhatia K. Unusual phenotypes in DYT1 dystonia: a report of five cases and a review of the literature. *Mov Disord*. 2003;18:706–11.

Gatto EM, Pardal MM, Micheli FE. Unusual phenotypic expression of the DYT1 mutation. *Parkinsonism Relat Disord*. 2003;9:277–9.

Video 17.1

There is a generalized dystonia with a superimposed jerky tremor, most evident in her upper limbs and neck. Her gait is dystonic and affected by superimposed jerks of her trunk.

Early Onset Generalized Dystonia with Cranio-Cervical Involvement: DYT6

Roberto Erro and Kailash P. Bhatia

Case 18

Clinical History

This 25-year-old woman noted having problems with her legs around the age of 7. Initially, her left leg was affected with plantar flexion of the foot, which made her walking awkwardly. Subsequently she found some difficulties with her handwriting and, at the age of 11 or 12 years, her speech became affected as well, because of her tongue involvement. Nevertheless, her eating and swallowing were preserved. After the initial worsening for about 5 years, she has then remained stable. From the point of view of her family history, her parents are first cousins and she has two siblings, all of whom are unaffected.

Examination

On examination (see Video 18.1), she had marked oromandibular dystonia with protrusion of the tongue. Her tongue also appeared to be somewhat hypertrophied and there was some prognathism of the jaw. There was generalized dystonia, with involvement of her arms, her trunk, and both feet, the left more than right. The feet dystonia was most evident on walking as the right hand dystonia was quite obvious on writing. The remaining neurological examination was unremarkable.

General Remarks

This woman presented with an isolated (formerly known as primary) dystonia which has affected her trunk, cranio-cervical region, and both lower and upper limbs (hence being generalized) with onset early in life. Given the long disease duration and the fact that she had a young-onset dystonia that then stabilized, the chances of her condition being "primary" dystonia, especially DYT6, are high (cf. Table 16.1). Nevertheless, the prominent oromandibular involvement might raise the suspicion of autosomal recessive forms of dystonia, also because there was a family history of consanguinity in her parents. However, in these forms

dystonia usually combines with other (neurological or not) system signs. The diagnostic work-up should be pursued accordingly. In this regard, a brain MRI to rule out brain iron accumulation as well as blood investigations for WD and neuroacanthocytosis, all of which can produce oromandibular dystonia, would be mandatory. Nevertheless, as stated earlier, none of these is likely, given the relatively paucity of symptoms beyond dystonia.

Investigations

Blood investigations, including copper and ceruloplasmin, as well as a brain MRI were normal. A genetic testing was pursued and she was found to carry the heterozygous variant c.C85T in exon 2 of *THAP1* gene, thus confirming a diagnosis of DYT6.

Special Remarks

THAP1-associated dystonia (DYT6) was first identified in three Mennonite families who were related by a common ancestor. Mutations in the *THAP1* gene account for up to 25 per cent of familial cases of early onset generalized dystonia. It is inherited in an autosomal dominant manner with penetrance estimated at 40 per cent. Some phenotypic features overlap with *TOR1A*-associated dystonia (DYT1), but the onset is usually later (mean is 24 years, with onset ranging from 2 to 62 years) and there is more prominent cranial involvement, especially in muscles of the larynx, and face, with dysphonia being a predominant feature. Besides the cranial involvement, there are differences between DYT6 and DYT1: the most common site of onset in the former is in fact the upper limb (47 per cent) followed by cranial dystonia (25 per cent), cervical dystonia (23 per cent), and rarely leg dystonia (17 per cent). Moreover, despite focal dystonia being described in DYT6 carriers, in more than half of them, dystonia spreads to become generalized or multifocal.

Management is basically based on anticholinergic drugs and/or botulinum toxin injections for the most affected sites. DBS of the globus pallidus is effective on long-term basis in patients with DYT6, even though the response rate is lower than in patients with DYT1.

Suggested Readings

Blanchard A, Ea V, Roubertie A, et al. DYT6 dystonia: review of the literature and creation of the UMD Locus-Specific Database (LSDB) for mutations in the THAP1 gene. *Hum Mutat*. 2011;32:1213–24.

Panov F, Tagliati M, Ozelius LJ, et al. Pallidal deep brain stimulation for DYT6 dystonia. *J Neurol Neurosurg Psychiatry*. 2012;83:182–7.

Xiromerisiou G, Houlden H, Scarmeas N, et al. THAP1 mutations and dystonia phenotypes: genotype phenotype correlations. *Mov Disord*. 2012;27:1290–4.

 Video 18.1

There is generalized dystonia with prominent oromandibular involvement and tongue enlargement. Dystonia is also seen in her arms, trunk, and lower limbs, particularly the left one.

Autosomal Recessive Isolated Generalized Dystonia: DYT2

Roberto Erro and Kailash P. Bhatia

Clinical History

This 58-year-old Sephardic Jewish man born from consanguineous healthy parents first developed abnormal postures of his left foot and leg at age 8 years. At the age of 12 years he also developed abnormal postures of the arms, difficulty writing, and an intermittent intention tremor. Over the following years he also developed torticollis and dysarthria, but had no significant progression since his late teenhood. He has two similarly affected siblings (Figure 19.1).

Examination

On examination (see Video 19.1), it was found he had generalized dystonia, most involving his cervical region and trunk. He also had facial grimacing, platysma overactivity, and a dystonic voice. There were dystonic movements of his head and arms on posture, with additional isolated non-stimulus-sensitive jerks. The abnormal posturing of his right arm was most evident on writing. His gait was dystonic. The remaining neurological examination was unremarkable.

General Remarks

This man presented early in his life with an isolated (formerly known as primary) generalized dystonia with no additional symptoms or signs but tremor. Given the long disease duration and the fact that he had a young-onset dystonia that then stabilized, the chances of his condition being "primary" dystonia are high. Given the consanguinity, one should consider recessive forms of isolated dystonia (cf. Table 16.1), although the fact that the proportion of affected siblings (3/3) is unusual. Conversely, dominant conditions with incomplete penetrance should also be considered.

Investigations

Extensive blood investigations (including those for secondary forms of dystonia) as well as a brain MRI were normal. Genetic testing for *TOR1A*, *THAP1*, *epsilon-sarcoglycan*, *GNAL*, and *ANO3* was inconclusive. With the use of a combination of homozygosity mapping and whole-exome sequencing, homozygous mutations (c.C225A) in exon 2 of the *HPCA* gene were found in this case as well as in his affected sisters, whereas their parents were found to be heterozygous carriers.

Special Remarks

Autosomal recessive forms of isolated dystonia have been previously lumped together under the rubric of DYT2 or 'DYT2-like' dystonia. The only genetically defined exception to this practice is with regard to DYT16, which is caused by homozygous mutation in the *PRKRA* gene. DYT16, however, most commonly presents with a phenotype of dystonia-parkinsonism, even though cases with pure dystonic syndromes have been rarely reported. Very recently, another recessive gene (e.g. *COL6A3* assigned to the DYT27 locus; Table 16.1) has been suggested – yet not confirmed – to cause early onset dystonia and should, therefore, be considered in the differential diagnosis.

DYT2 was first reported in three families of consanguineous Spanish gypsies, but the diagnosis remained equivocal since DYT2 was simply defined by the phenotype of isolated generalized dystonia and by its recessive mode of inheritance rather than by an association with a specific genetic locus. 'Sephardic' is derived from Hebrew for 'Spain' and refers to the descendants of a large Jewish community living in Spain and Portugal in the Middle Ages. Therefore, this might indicate a higher prevalence of DYT2 in this ethnic group.

The *HPCA* gene encodes hippocalcin, a protein highly expressed in the striatum, the function of which suggests a role for perturbed calcium signaling in the pathogenesis of this condition.

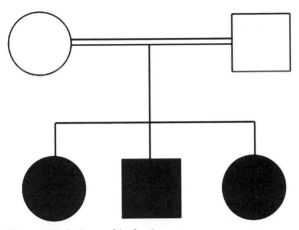

Figure 19.1 Pedigree of the family.

Domingo A, Erro R, Lohmann K. Novel dystonia genes: clues on disease mechanisms and the complexities of high-throughput sequencing. *Mov Disord.* 2016;31:471–7.

Khan NL, Wood NW, Bhatia KP. Autosomal recessive, DYT2-like primary torsion dystonia – a new family. *Neurology.* 2003;61:1801–3.

 Video 19.1

There is generalized dystonia, mainly involving his cervical region and trunk. He also has facial grimacing and platysma overactivity. There are dystonic movements of his head and arms on posture, with an additional jerking component. The abnormal posturing of his right arm can be best appreciated on writing.

Suggested Readings

Charlesworth G, Angelova PR, Bartolomé-Robledo F, et al. Mutations in HPCA cause autosomal-recessive primary isolated dystonia. *Am J Hum Genet.* 2015;96:657-65.

Dopa-Responsive Dystonia

Roberto Erro and Kailash P. Bhatia

Clinical History

This 17-year-old man presented at a young age with developmental delay; he was able to crawl only at 18 months. He did not walk independently until 19 months and continued to have frequent falls. There was also speech delay. He was diagnosed with cerebral palsy, but at age 3, he was given a trial of levodopa, which dramatically improved his symptoms. At the age of 12, the levodopa was discontinued and he again developed limping and falling, confirming that he had a sort of DRD, which could be better on some days than others, being particularly worse when there is cold weather. Over his childhood and adolescence, he managed to attend normal school and is now completely independent.

As to his family history, his father was diagnosed with hemiplegic cerebral palsy and epilepsy.

Examination

On examination (see Video 20.1), he had a rather fixed dystonia of his left foot, which was in-turned, and affected his walking. Apart from a mild abnormal posturing in his upper limbs, the remaining neurological examination was normal.

General Remarks

This young man presented with an isolated dystonic syndrome starting at a very young age with minimal progression. Given his response to levodopa, a suspicion of DRD very high and, in this context, it is possible that his father was misdiagnosed with hemiplegic cerebral palsy. Given the benign phenotype, the autosomal dominant form of DRD (or Segawa disease) is most likely, being the recessive ones (cf. Case 21) more severe, usually complicated by other symptoms/signs and only partially responsive to levodopa. The diagnostic work-up should be performed to prove a deficit in the dopamine biosynthesis pathway (Figure 20.1), and a CSF evaluation for dopamine metabolites and

pterins should be the first approach to subsequently lead the genetic analyses.

Investigations and Diagnosis

CSF examination showed reduced BH4, HVA, and 5-HIAA values, thus supporting GCH1 deficiency (Figure 20.1). Genetic testing of the *GCH1* gene confirmed that he carried an intronic c.353+5G>C mutation, likely affecting *GCH1* splicing, and thus confirming a diagnosis of DRD (Segawa variant).

Special Remarks

Segawa first reported nine patients in six families with dystonic posturing showing marked diurnal fluctuation. Dystonic posture or movement of one limb appeared between ages 1 and 9 years. All limbs were eventually involved within 5 years of onset in a subset of patients, while trunk involvement was unusual. Described in general, the majority of patients classically have one or both legs affected after several years from onset. Rigidity, resting tremor, or cerebellar, pyramidal, and sensory changes were not found, and cognition was normal. Symptoms were remarkably alleviated after sleep and aggravated gradually towards evening and showed a dramatic response to levodopa treatment. However, after the discovery of *GCH1* mutations as causative of the condition described by Segawa, it has become clear that patients can additionally present with parkinsonian signs, including tremor and slowness, especially if the onset is later in life. Moreover, approximately one-quarter of patients also have hyperreflexia, particularly in the legs.

The *GCH1* gene encodes the rate-limiting enzyme for the synthesis of tetrahydrobiopterin (BH4), an essential cofactor for the conversion of tyrosine to levodopa (Figure 20.1), thus explaining the striking therapeutic response. Levodopa is in fact the most effective treatment, and patients exhibit an excellent

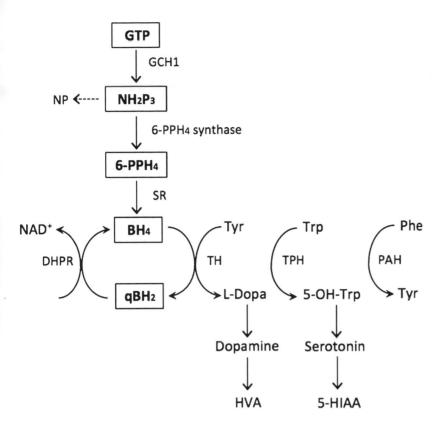

Figure 20.1 Pterins and dopamine pathway.
(GTP: Guanosine-5-triphosphate; GCH1: GTP cyclohydrolase 1; NH$_2$P$_3$: Dihydroneopterin triphosphate; NP: Neopterin; 6-PPH$_4$: 6-Pyrovoyl-tetrahydropterin; SR: Sepiapterin reductase; BH$_4$: Tetrahydrobiopterin; qBH$_2$: q-Dihydrobiopterin; DHPR: dihydropteridine reductase; NAD: Nicotinamide adenine dinucleotide; Tyr: Tyrosine; TH: Tyrosine hydroxylase; HVA: homovanillic acid; Trp: Tryptophan; TPH: Tryptophan hydroxylase; 5-OH-Trp: 5-hydroxytryptophan; 5 HIAA: 5-hydroxyindoleacetic acid; Phe: Phenylalanine; PAH: Phenylalanine hydroxylase.)

response to low doses (usually between 100 and 300 mg daily) lasting as long as 25 years. Yet, residual motor signs while patients are on treatment are possible. These might not necessarily interfere with the patients' daily activities but are easily detectable on examination. More recently, it has also become clear that patients with DRD might have higher frequencies of depression, anxiety, and obsessive-compulsive disorder as compared with the general population.

The dramatic responsiveness to levodopa clearly differentiates DRD from other forms of idiopathic torsion dystonia that have a similar phenotype. In addition, the sustained nature of the levodopa responsiveness with absence in most of the cases of levodopa-induced dyskinesias distinguishes DRD (also known as DYT5a; cf. Table 16.1) from other causes of childhood-onset dystonia-parkinsonism or early onset parkinsonian syndromes. In this regard, CSF investigation is crucial for the differential diagnosis since it is generally normal in all other conditions of dystonia-parkinsonism or early onset parkinsonism. Alternatively, the phenylalanine loading test can be useful to aid the differential diagnosis, even though its sensitivity seems to be rather

low. The basis for this test is that BH4 is required as a cofactor in the breakdown of phenylalanine to tyrosine. Therefore, in DRD, BH4 deficiency results in the accumulation of phenylalanine.

Suggested Readings
Segawa M. Dopa-responsive dystonia. *Handb Clin Neurol.* 2011;100:539–57.

Tadic V, Kasten M, Brüggemann N, Stiller S, Hagenah J, Klein C. Dopa-responsive dystonia revisited: diagnostic delay, residual signs, and nonmotor signs. *Arch Neurol.* 2012;69:1558–62.

Wijemanne S, Jankovic J. Dopa-responsive dystonia- clinical and genetic heterogeneity. *Nat Rev Neurol.* 2015;11:414–24

 Video 20.1

This patient has a left foot dystonia, which is turned inwards and affects his walking. Note the callosity on the outer margin of the foot. There is mild dystonia in his upper limbs.

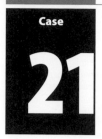

Case

21

A Complicated Dopa-Responsive Dystonia: Tyrosine Hydroxylase Deficiency

Roberto Erro and Kailash P. Bhatia

Clinical History

This 19-year-old girl, born from consanguineous parents, has had severe developmental delay since birth and never achieved milestones, not being able to sit up, crawl, stand, or walk. Early in her childhood, she progressively developed generalized dystonia, which was most evident in the upper limbs. She also started having paroxysmal events with further abnormal posturing, which were first interpreted as seizures, despite the absence of clear EEG correlates and, in fact, trials with different antiepileptics were proven unhelpful. A trial of L-dopa was subsequently performed and this led to a consistent, albeit partial, improvement with regard to both the generalized dystonia and the paroxysmal events.

Examination

The examination (see Video 21.1) was limited due to significant mental delay. She had a dystonic posturing of the neck, both hands with flexion at wrist and extension of fingers and slight eversion of the feet. There were few facial twitches along with non-stimulus-sensitive, spontaneous myoclonic jerks in both upper and lower limbs. Occasional choreoathetoid movements could also be detected in the upper limbs. Hypokinesia was noted on finger tapping. She was wheelchair bound and could not stand or walk unaided, also due to the presence of truncal hypothonia. She could not articulate any words or sentences, but could repeat short phonemes, her speech appearing hypophonic and dysarthric. Finger–nose testing was normal. The deep tendon jerks were brisk in all limbs.

General Remarks

This complex syndrome with generalized dystonia, parkinsonian features, and developmental delay is not usually seen in inherited isolated dystonic syndromes (formerly known as primary) and would suggest secondary causes. As such, a wide number of different disorders should be considered in the differential diagnosis, and the diagnostic work-up should be performed accordingly (cf. Table 22.1). However, the response to L-dopa, albeit partial, narrows the differential diagnosis to the DRD syndromes. DRD syndromes are a group of disorders that represent about 5 per cent of childhood dystonias. The autosomal dominant form due to *GCH1* mutations is most common (cf. Case 20) and is the most benign, typically showing an excellent and sustained response to low doses of L-dopa. On the contrary, two autosomal recessive forms of DRD have been identified: TH deficiency and sepiapterin reductase deficiency, both usually less responsive to L-dopa and often accompanied by intellectual disability and ocular abnormalities such as oculogyric crisis, upwards gaze, and ptosis. CSF examination is most useful to aid the differential diagnosis. Finally, there are other two rare disorders that can produce similar phenotypes and are associated with deficits in the neurotransmitter transporting system rather than in the dopamine biosynthesis pathway. Mutations of *SLC6A3* result in dopamine transporter (DaT) deficiency. For the diagnosis, DaT-Scan imaging is very helpful, revealing complete loss or a severe reduction of DaT binding in the basal ganglia. Vesicular monoamine transporter 2 (VAMT2) deficiency due to mutations in *SLC18A2* affects several neurotransmitter systems (i.e. dopamine, serotonin, epinephrine, and norepinephrine). This disorder can share many clinical features with complicated DRD syndromes, although L-dopa is far less effective. CSF examination shows normal neurotransmitter levels.

Investigations and Diagnosis

An extensive diagnostic work-up revealed no blood or imaging (including DaT-Scan) abnormalities. On the contrary, CSF examination showed reduced HVA and normal 5-HIAA values, with reduced HVA/5-HIAA ratio and normal BH4 levels, thus supporting the diagnosis of TH deficiency (cf. Figure 20.1), which was subsequently genetically confirmed.

Special Remarks

TH deficiency is a rare autosomal recessive disorder that can be associated with a wide phenotypic spectrum. Based on the symptom severity and responsiveness to L-dopa therapy, three main phenotypes have been recognized and, from mildest to most severe, they are: TH-deficient dopa-responsive dystonia (also referred to as DYT5b); TH-deficient infantile parkinsonism with motor delay; and TH-deficient progressive infantile encephalopathy. However, several atypical severe forms have been recognized and this was the case in our patient, who presented with developmental delay and generalized dystonia.

In DRD due to *TH* mutations, onset of symptoms is between ages 12 months and 6 years, and the initial symptoms are usually represented by lower limb dystonia and/or difficulty in walking. In general, gradual progression to generalized dystonia occurs. Bradykinesia and tremor (mainly postural) can be observed, as well as features suggestive of pyramidal signs (hyperreflexia, increased tone, and/or extensor plantar responses). There is also a tendency to fall. Intellect is not impaired in individuals with this form of TH deficiency. In rare instances, sustained upward ocular deviations (oculogyric crises) are observed. Diurnal fluctuation of symptoms has been reported in up to 30 per cent of TH-deficient DRD cases, a much lower estimate than observed in DRD due to *GCH1* mutations.

In the severe form of TH deficiency, onset is between ages 3 and 12 months with motor delay and severe parkinsonism. In contrast to TH-deficient DRD, motor milestones are overtly delayed and often there is mental retardation as well. Virtually all affected individuals demonstrate truncal hypotonia as well as additional parkinsonian features. Moreover, oculogyric crises are often observed and ptosis and features of mild autonomic dysfunction can be present. Despite dystonia being almost invariably present, it tends to be less prominent, and typical diurnal fluctuation of symptoms is not observed in most patients with TH-deficient infantile parkinsonism with motor delay.

Interestingly, diurnal variation of axial hypotonia but not of limb dystonia has been described.

The most severe form of TH deficiency has neonatal-onset, and affected individuals demonstrate feeding difficulties, hypotonia, and/or retarded somatic parameters (head circumference, height, and/or weight) from birth. Moreover, there can be severe hypokinesia, limb hypertonia (rigidity and/or spasticity), hyperreflexia with extensor plantar responses, oculogyric crises, bilateral ptosis, and paroxysmal periods of lethargy (with increased sweating) that alternated with irritability (so-called lethargy-irritability crises). Individuals with TH-deficient progressive infantile encephalopathy are extremely sensitive to L-dopa, often developing intolerable dyskinesias at the initiation of the therapy.

Despite the clear recognition of these three phenotypes, no phenotype–genotype correlations have been elucidated. There has been a suggestion that timing of L-dopa introduction would influence the long-term outcomes, at least as far as the mildest forms are concerned, and therefore prompt diagnosis of TH deficiency is crucial.

Suggested Readings

de Rijk-van Andel JF, Gabreels FJM, Geurtz B, et al. L-dopa-responsive infantile hypokinetic rigid parkinsonism due to tyrosine hydroxylase deficiency. *Neurology*. 2000;55:1926–8.

Lee WW, Jeon BS. Clinical spectrum of dopa-responsive dystonia and related disorders. *Curr Neurol Neurosci Rep*. 2014;14:461.

Willemsen MA, Verbeek MM, Kamsteeg EJ, et al. Tyrosine hydroxylase deficiency: a treatable disorder of brain catecholamine biosynthesis. *Brain*. 2010;133:1810–22.

 Video 21.1

This patient has spontaneous myoclonic jerks in her face and both upper and lower limbs. There is a clear dysarthria, and dystonia is most evident in her neck and upper limbs. She is slow bilaterally on finger tapping. Unaided walking is impossible: her gait is impaired due to the presence of dystonic features in the lower limbs and truncal hypothonia.

Early Onset Generalized Dystonia and Macrocephaly: Glutaric Aciduria Type 1

Roberto Erro and Kailash P. Bhatia

Clinical History

This 24-year-old man was born from consanguineous parents (first cousins) and started having problems in his early infancy. He was found to be macrocephalic, and his early milestones were delayed, with an inability to sit, stand, or walk. He never managed to walk independently and has been wheelchair bound for all his life, using a foam carved insert to support his trunk being still. He also developed dystonic spasms in his first year of life, which worsened over time, and are currently so severe that he is highly dependent for any day-to-day activities. In addition, he developed speech and swallowing difficulties early in the disease course, which were also progressive and in fact, his speech is now quite hard to understand and he has lost 4 pounds over the last year. More recently, he also developed episodes of nocturnal distress.

Examination

On examination (see Video 22.1), he was in a wheelchair, not being able to stand and walk. He had macrocephaly and his speech was grossly dysarthric, with dystonia being the main component. He showed generalized dystonia, which has also affected the cranial region and the tongue. A fixed contracture of his left hand was seen and he could not use it at all. Limbs were hypotonic at rest. When he attempted voluntary movements, dyskinetic movements in the contralateral limbs could also be elicited. Other findings on examination included weakness of all four limbs (left>right) with brisk reflexes, while cerebellar examination was normal.

General Remarks

As discussed in Case 21, a complex syndrome featuring delayed milestones and generalized dystonia with superimposed bulbar and pyramidal symptoms would not fit in with a 'primary' dystonic syndrome

and would rather suggest a secondary cause. Also, given the very early age at onset and clinical progression, an acquired cause would be unlikely. In such cases, the diagnostic work-up is rather wide and should hence comprise a number of tests (mainly on blood and urine) to exclude inborn error of metabolism, some of which are treatable disorders (Table 22.1). Obviously, other conditions should be considered if the biochemical investigations come back all normal, thus excluding organic acidurias and lysosomal storage disorders. There was, however, a clinical clue (i.e. macrocephaly) that could have helped reaching the diagnosis. In this context, in fact, the association of delayed milestones, generalized dystonia, macrocephaly, and encephalopathic crises makes the diagnosis of Glutaric Aciduria type 1 most likely.

Investigations and Diagnosis

Urinary organic acid evaluation showed very increased glutaric (1058 mcmol/mmol creatinine) and high 3-hydroxyglutaric acid (42 mcmol/mmol creatinine), which were suggestive of Glutaric Aciduria type 1. Brain MRI (Figure 22.1), beyond an altered cranial-facial ratio indicating macrocrania, showed prominence of the extra-axial spaces over the cerebral hemispheres mainly involving the bilateral sylvian and perisylvian regions, worse on the right side. Furthermore, there were bilateral and symmetrical signal abnormalities and volume loss involving the putamina and, to a lesser extent, the genu of the corpus callosum. Moderate to severe subcortical volume loss was also seen in the cerebral white matter, more severe in a centripetal distribution. Furthermore, there was evidence of a previous subdural haemorrhage over the left fronto-temporal convex. Genetic testing for the *GCDH* gene, encoding glutaryl-CoA dehydrogenase, confirmed that he was homozygous for the c.C298T mutation in exon 3, thus confirming the diagnosis of Glutaric Aciduria type 1.

Table 22.1 Useful Biochemical Investigations to Identify Inborn Errors of Metabolism that May Present with Dystonia

Sample(s)	Laboratory test(s)	Disorder(s)
Urine	Organic acids	Glutaric Aciduria type 1, propionic aciduria, methylmalonic aciduria, cobalamin deficiencies
Plasma	Lactate	Propionic aciduria, methylmalonic aciduria, biotin responsive basal ganglia disease
Plasma	Pyruvate	Pyruvate dehydrogenase complex deficiency
Plasma	Acylcarnitines	Glutaric Aciduria type 1, propionic aciduria, methylmalonic aciduria
Plasma	Amino acids	Ornithine transcarbamylase deficiency, maple syrup urine disease, pterin defects
Plasma	Homocysteine	Homocystinuria
Plasma/Urine	Copper, Ceruloplasmin	Wilson's disease
Plasma	Manganese	Dystonia with brain manganese accumulation (*SLC30A10* mutations)
Plasma	Biotinidase	Biotinidase deficiency
Plasma/Urine	Creatine, guanidinoacetic acid	Cerebral creatine deficiency syndrome 3, guanidinoacetate methyltransferase deficiency
Plasma	Vitamine E	Ataxia with vitamine E deficiency
Plasma	Uric acid	Lesch–Nyhan syndrome
Plasma	Cholestanol	Cerebrotendinous xanthomatosis
Plasma/CSF	Glucose	GLUT-1 deficiency
CSF	Folate	Cerebral folate deficiency
CSF	Pterins, dopamine and serotonin metabolites	GTP-cyclohydrolase 1 deficiency, Tyrosine hydroxylase deficiency, Sepiapterin reductase deficiency, 6-pyruvoyl-tetrahydropterin synthase deficiency, aromatic l-amino acid decarboxylase deficiency

Source: Modified from van Egmond, Kuiper A, Eggink H, et al. 2014.

Special Remarks

Glutaric Aciduria type 1 is a rare (estimated prevalence of 1 in 100,000 newborns), autosomal recessive, inborn error of metabolism due to deficiency of a flavin adenine dinucleotide-dependent mitochondrial matrix protein (glutaryl-CoA dehydrogenase), which is involved in the degradative metabolism of L-lysine, L-hydroxylysine, and L-tryptophan. Four genetic isolates with a high carrier (up to 1:10) and affected individual frequency have been identified: the Amish Community, the Canadian Oji-Cree natives, the Irish travellers, and the Lumbee in North Carolina.

Biochemically, Glutaric Aciduria type 1 is characterized by an accumulation of glutaric and 3-hydroxyglutaric acid, and less frequently glutaconic acid and glutarylcarnitine. Two biochemically defined subgroups of patients have been described based on urinary metabolite excretion (i.e. low and high excretors), but the low excreting patients have been deemed to have the same risk of developing neurological symptoms and striatal injury as the high excretors. They

should not hence be considered to be less prone to develop a severe clinical phenotype.

Untreated, almost all patients develop neurological symptoms within 36 months of life, usually following an acute encephalopathic crisis often precipitated by gastroenteritis, intercurrent febrile illness, immunization, or surgical intervention. The classical neurological involvement encompasses an acute bilateral striatal injury followed by a complex movement disorder, where dystonia is the dominant feature, usually superimposed on axial hypotonia. With aging, there is a tendency for fixed dystonic contractures and akinetic-rigid parkinsonism to develop. In a summary, this disorder includes macrocephaly (up to 75 per cent of patients), acute encephalopathy, basal ganglia injury, white matter disease, movement disorders, and subdural and retinal hemorrhage.

More than 200 mutations have been reported to date, but there is no clear genotype–phenotype correlation and in fact some patients might have a more benign clinical picture (Video 22.2). Glutaric Aciduria type 1 is now considered to be a treatable condition,

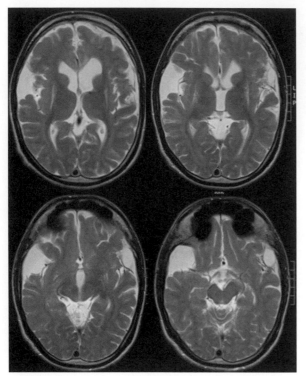

Figure 22.1 Axial T2 sequences showing prominence of the extra-axial spaces over the cerebral hemispheres, in particular involving the bilateral sylvian and perisylvian regions, are worse on the right side. There are bilateral and symmetrical signal abnormalities and volume loss involving the putamina. Moderate to severe subcortical volume loss is seen in the cerebral white matter and more severe in a centripetal distribution.

and most patients remain asymptomatic if treatment is started in the newborn period. For this reason, Glutaric Aciduria type 1 has been included in the disease panel of newborn screening in some countries. Managment consists of low-lysine diet in combination with carnitine and emergency treatments for

intercurrent encephalopathic crises. This combination has been demonstrated to be effective in preventing neurological disability. The outcome is in fact better in patients who receive all three types of interventions. Conversely, outcome is poor when the diagnosis (and treatment) is made after the onset of neurological symptoms.

Suggested Readings

Kölker S, Christensen E, Leonard JV, et al. Diagnosis and management of glutaric aciduria type I revised recommendations. *J Inherit Metab Dis.* 2011;34(3):677–94.

van Egmond ME, Kuiper A, Eggink H, et al. Dystonia in children and adolescents: a systematic review and a new diagnostic algorithm. *J Neurol Neurosurg Psychiatry.* 2015;86:774–81.

Video 22.1

This patient is in a wheelchair and is not able to stand and walk. He has macrocephaly and his speech is grossly dysarthric, with dystonia being the main component. He has generalized dystonia, which has affected the cranial region and the tongue. A fixed contracture of his left hand is seen and he could not use it at all; there is also evidence of mild weakness.

Video 22.2

This patient with Glutaric Aciduria type 1 has a mild phenotype with hemi-dystonia that has affected the right side of his body and additional pyramidal signs in his right leg.

23

PKAN Misdiagnosed as 'Progressive Delayed-Onset Postanoxic Dystonia'

Roberto Erro and Kailash P. Bhatia

Clinical History

This 50-year-old woman with no family history for any neurological disorders suffered a cardiac arrest at the age of 19 during induction of general anesthesia for a minor dental surgery. After resuscitation, she was comatose for 48 hours but recovered afterwards and was hence discharged home a week later without residual deficits. A few months later, she started having writing difficulty with abnormal posturing and micrographia. She was also found to have speech articulation problems. These symptoms were progressive and about 2 years later she also developed right leg dystonia. At this stage, she was diagnosed with postanoxic dystonia and was told that a further progression would have been unlikely. Nevertheless, she continued to worsen over the years, with particular regard of her gait, speech, and swallowing. Her first brain MRI was performed at the age of 24 (5 years later than clinical onset) and showed bilateral T2 hypointensities in globus pallidus, suggestive of mineral accumulation. While a CT scan excluded calcifications, the overall appearance was claimed to be consistent with anoxic injury, possibly related to hemorrhagic transformation associated with anoxia. Yet her clinical picture continued to deteriorate and by the age of 35 a gastrostomy tube was inserted, whilst an emergency tracheotomy was done at 43 years of age (24 years after symptom onset), following recurrent episodes of stridor.

Examination

Facial expression was hypomimic with additional dystonic grimace and there was prominent 'jaw-opening' oromandibular dystonia (Video 23.1). Tongue movements were very slow and she was completely anarthric. There was generalized dystonia, affecting her lower limbs more than the upper ones. Rapid alternating movements of the hands were suggestive of bradykinesia. She also had pyramidal signs, namely brisk reflexes in the lower limbs with bilateral extensor plantar responses. Gait was possible for brief distances, but was dystonic and severely affected by loss of postural reflexes.

General Remarks

Although delayed onset of dystonia after hypoxic–ischemic events is a well-known phenomenon, especially in children and young adults, such a dramatic progression over a very long period of more than 20 years with further development of dysphagia (requiring a gastrostomy tube) and severe stridor episodes (requiring an emergency tracheotomy) was very unusual and suggested another cause. Such a severe phenotype of generalized dystonia with prominent oromandibular involvement (usually of the 'jaw-opening' type) and swallowing difficulties is normally not seen in 'primary' forms and should prompt to look for secondary heredodegenerative causes.

Investigations and Diagnosis

A brain MRI scan showed bilateral pallidal hypointensity on T2 sequences, suggestive of iron accumulation (Figure 23.1A). SWI sequences confirmed excessive iron accumulation with the lobus pallidus bilaterally (Figure 23.1B). Direct DNA sequencing for the *PANK2* gene was therefore performed and she was found to be compound heterozygote for c.498_499delITG and c.T563A mutations in the exon 2, thus leading to a definite diagnosis of PKAN.

Special Remarks

PKAN (also referred to as NBIA1 and formerly known as Hallervorden–Spatz disease) is an autosomal recessive disorder due to *PANK2* mutations, with estimated prevalence of 1–3:1,000,000, thus accounting for the majority of NBIA cases (up to 50 per cent, Table 23.1). Since the discovery of its genetic underpinnings in 2001, two main phenotypes have been delineated. Classic PKAN has an onset in the first decade, usually

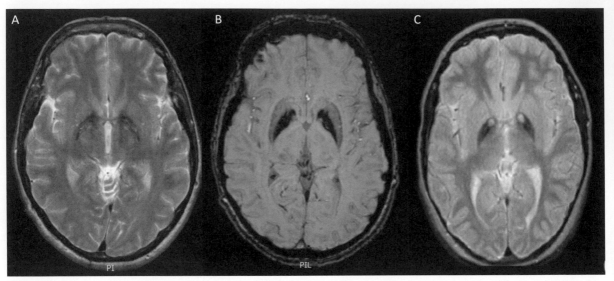

Figure 23.1 Axial T2 (A) and SWI (B) sequences showing iron accumulation within the globus pallidus bilaterally, while the typical 'eye of the tiger' sign is shown in (C).

Table 23.1 Overview of the NBIA Syndromes

Condition/Acronym	Synonym	Gene (chromosomal position)	Inheritance	MRI pattern
PKAN	NBIA1	*PANK2* (20p13)	AR	'Eye of the tiger' sign
PLAN*	NBIA2, NAD, INAD, PARK14	*PLA2G6* (22q12)	AR	T2 hypointensity globus pallidus, white matter hyperintensity, cerebellar atrophy,
Neuroferritinopathy	NBIA3	*FTL* (19q13)	AD	T2 hypointensity globus pallidus, putamen, and/or thalamus (with patchy involvement). Possible hyperintensity (cavitation) with the pallidus
MPAN	NBIA4	*C19orf12* (19q12)	AR	T2 hypointensity in the globus pallidus and substantia nigra. T2 hyperintense streaking of the medial medullary lamina between the globus pallidus interna and externa. Cortical and cerebellar atrophy can be seen.
BPAN	NBIA5	*WDR45 (Xp11.23)*	X-linked (dominant)	T2 hypointensity in the globus pallidus and substantia nigra; T1 hyperintensity of the substantia nigra with a central band of hypointensity
CoPAN	NBIA6	*COASY* (17q12)	AR	T2 hypointensity in the globus pallidus and substantia nigra and mild hyperintensity in the caudate, putamen and posterior thalamus
Aceruloplasminemia	–	*CP* (3q23)	AR	Simultaneous and confluent involvement of basal ganglia and cortex; white matter hyperintensity; cerebellar atrophy

Table 23.1 (continued)

Condition/Acronym	Synonym	Gene (chromosomal position)	Inheritance	MRI pattern
FHAN	–	*FA2H (16q23)*	AR	T2 hypointensity in the basal ganglia, midbrain and cerebellar atrophy
Kufor-Rakeb*	PARK9	*ATP13A2* (1p36.13)	AR	T2 hypointensity in the globus pallidus and cortical atrophy
Woodhouse-Sakati*	–	*C2ORF37* (2q31.1)	AR	T2 hypointensity in the basal ganglia and white matter hyperintensity

* Iron accumulation may be absent on imaging.
Abb.: AR: Autosomal recessive; AD: Autosomal dominant; NAD: Neuroaxonal Dystrophy; INAD: Infantile Neuroaxonal Dystrophy; MPAN: Mitochondrial membrane protein-associated neurodegeneration; BPAN: Beta-propeller protein-associated neurodegeneration; CoPAN: COASY Protein-Associated Neurodegeneration; FHAN: Fatty Acid Hydroxylase-Associated Neurodegeneration.

with gait and balance problems and a rapid progression leading to loss of ambulation within 10–15 years. Onset of atypical PKAN is in the second or third decade, often with dystonia with prominent oromandibular and/or trunk involvement. The phenotype is almost invariably complicated by the presence of bulbar symptoms, but the progression is slower, with loss of mobility after 15–40 years. Iron accumulation within the globus pallidus bilaterally (manifesting as hypointensity on T2 sequences or – even better – on dedicated sequence including SWI and gradient-echo T2*) is invariably present and may even predate the clinical symptoms. There is often an additional central focus of increased signal (reflecting edema and gliosis) and, in such case, the overall appearance has been referred to as 'eye of the tiger' sign (Figure 23.1C). The 'eye of the tiger' sign has been deemed to be pathognomonic of PKAN, but its absence (like in our case) does not exclude *PANK2* mutations. Hence, the diagnosis should not rely solely on this sign, since it may be absent both early and very late in the disease course.

Unfortunately, there is no efficacious treatment and management should be pursued empirically. More recently, clinical trials with Deferiprone, an iron chelator agent, have been performed which yielded preliminary promising results. On the contrary, there is an increased interest in DBS of the globus pallidus internus as a symptomatic treatment option for dystonia in PKAN, the response being, however, highly variable with decreasing efficacy over time. Despite there being no reliable prognostic factors regarding DBS outcomes in these patients, it may be a life-saving procedure in patients with status dystonicus not responding to oral medications.

Suggested Readings

Kruer MC, Boddaert N, Schneider SA, et al. Neuroimaging features of neurodegeneration with brain iron accumulation. *AJNR Am J Neuroradiol.* 2012;33:407–14.

Schneider SA, Hardy J, Bhatia KP. Syndromes of neurodegeneration with brain iron accumulation (NBIA): an update on clinical presentations, histological and genetic underpinnings, and treatment considerations. *Mov Disord.* 2012;27:42–53.

 Video 23.1

Prominent jaw-opening dystonia is shown. There is additional (mild) dystonic posturing in the upper limbs, where a postural tremor also occurs. Ocular movements on the vertical plane are restricted. Gait reflects a combination of dystonic and spastic features.

24 Oromandibular Dystonia and Freezing of Gait: A Novel Presentation of Neuroferritinopathy

Roberto Erro and Kailash P. Bhatia

Clinical History

This 37-year-old young woman presented with an 18-month history of difficulties with her left arm and speech symptoms. She mentioned that her symptoms began when she was pregnant with her fourth child, having developed high blood pressure and pre-eclampsia. Around this time, she noticed that her speech was affected. Moreover, she tended to clench her jaw and her teeth were grinding together. A trial with botulinum toxin injections into the masseter muscles to relieve her jaw clenching was proven unhelpful and she found that keeping a piece of cotton wool in her mouth would reduce the jaw movements. Shortly after, she developed swallowing difficulties and was noted to choke on liquids. Moreover, her left arm and hand started twisting and she also experienced walking difficulties. No other subjective complaints were reported, but her mother mentioned that she not as sharp as she was used to be.

Examination

On examination (see Video 24.1) it was found that she had very clear oromandibular dystonia, with jaw-closing spasms, side-to-side jaw movements and additional choreic features. Furthermore, she had motor impersistence when protruding her tongue and was found to be dysarthric, with dystonic features being the main component. She had frontalis hyperactivity, but ocular movements were full and normal. There was abnormal posturing and athetoid movements in her upper limbs, both at rest and on posture. She had difficulties with finger tapping, particularly on the left side, but no true fatiguing. She showed marked freezing of gait on turning and postural reflexes loss. Otherwise, her examination was normal.

General Remarks

The prominent abnormality in this case is that of severe oromandibular dystonia. In general, pronounced oromandibular dystonia characterized by involuntary movements of muscles of the lower face, mouth, and tongue would be uncommon in primary dystonia and rather suggests a secondary (i.e. tardive) or heredodegenerative form of dystonia, mainly including NBIA syndromes, neuroacanthocytosis, and Lesch–Nyhan syndrome. Moreover, the presence of additional findings on examination, including walking and balance difficulties, would not fit with a 'primary' (isolated and idiopathic) ormandibular dystonia, which usually presents later in life, has a much slower progression, and does not classically encompass other neurological symptoms besides dystonia.

The absence of secondary causes such as exposure to neuroleptic drugs and/or hypoxic/anoxic events pointed towards a heredodegenerative form of dystonia.

Investigations and Diagnosis

Basic serum investigations, including screening for acanthocytes on three serial films, were all normal. A brain MRI showed bilateral, fairly symmetrical signal abnormalities and some volume changes in the lentifrom nuclei. Notably, T2 hypointensity was noted in the globi pallidi, within which there were areas of hyperintense on T2 (Figure 24.1), suggesting the presence of the 'eye of the tiger' sign (cf. Case 24). However, on SWI sequences further areas of increased hypointensity were seen in the pallidostriatal pathway, red nuclei, dentate nuclei, and to a lesser extent in the thalamic nuclei and the putamina (Figure 24.2). In addition, the cortical outline of both cerebral hemispheres and cerebellum was exaggerated (again due to the increased susceptibility due to mineral deposition). Altogether, imaging findings were supportive of NBIA. Although the 'eye of the tiger' was suggested, the topographical distribution of iron accumulation, including cortical sulci lining (along with the 'late' age at onset), prompted us to screen her for neuroferritinopathy first. A 1bp

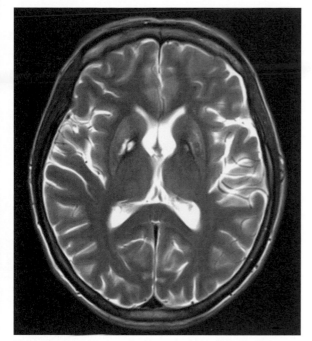

Figure 24.1 MRI T2-weigthed sequences showing a pseudo- 'eye of the tiger' sign.

duplication in exon 4 of the ferritin light chain gene (*FTL* c.460dupA) on chromosome 19 was detected, confirming the diagnosis of neuroferritinopathy.

Special Remarks

Neuroferritinopathy (also labeled as NBIA type 2; cf. Table 23.1) is the only autosomal dominant NBIA syndrome described to date, the onset of which is in adulthood (mean age of onset: 39 years). Its main clinical features are that of movement disorders, with chorea (50 per cent) being the most common presentation, followed by focal dystonia (43 per cent) and parkinsonism (7.5 per cent). Patients often have a typical facies with activated frontalis muscles and usually have bulbar involvement with dysarthria and swallowing difficulties early in the disease. Moreover, subsequent development of oro-buccal dyskinesias and slow tongue movement, along with stereotypical tapping movements, are characteristic clinical findings in this disease. Cognition is deemed to be grossly spared, even though mild cognitive and neuropsychiatric dysfunction can occur. The disease progresses over time and signs can change from side to side, namely patients can develop rigidity in limbs where they previously had choreiform movements and vice versa.

Besides brain MR imaging, low serum ferritin levels are supportive of the diagnosis. Although serum ferritin levels have been reported to be decreased in up to 80 per cent of males and all post-menopausal females, about 75 per cent of pre-menopausal females

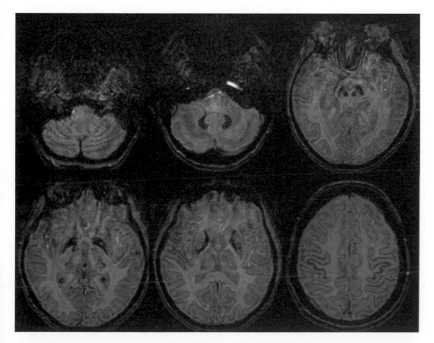

Figure 24.2 MRI SWI-sequences showing signal of high susceptibility (suggesting iron accumulation) within the pallidostriatal pathway, red nuclei, dentate nuclei in the cortical outline of both cerebral hemispheres and cerebellum.

have normal serum ferritin values (as in our case). The topography of brain iron accumulation can aid the differential diagnosis among NBIA syndromes. In neuroferritinopathy, excess iron deposition becomes evident in the putamen, globus pallidus, and dentate nucleus, with a 'patchy' distribution. The caudate and thalamus may also be involved. Cystic cavitation evolves with time and may be preceded by hyperintense T1-weighted signal intensity, particularly in the putamen and globus pallidus, thus generating the potential for a pseudo 'eye of the tiger' sign. More recently, the 'cortical pencil lining' sign, reflecting abnormal iron deposition at the cortical level, has been suggested as a diagnostic clue for neuroferritinopathy.

No treatment exists for this condition and no medication has been found to date to influence disease progression, including iron chelating therapy. Treatment is mainly symptomatic, according to the main clinical presentation.

Suggested Readings

Batla A, Adams M, Erro R, et al. Cortical pencil lining in neuroferritinopathy: a diagnostic clue. *Neurology*. 2015;84:1816–18.

Chinnery PF, Crompton DE, Birchall D, et al. Clinical features and natural history of neuroferritinopathy caused by the FTL1 460InsA mutation. *Brain*. 2007;130:110–9.

Lehn A, Boyle R, Brown H, Airey C, Mellick G. Neuroferritinopathy. *Parkinsonism Relat Disord*. 2012;18:909–15.

 Video 24.1

This patient has oromandibular dyskinesia with motor impersistence when asked to protrude her tongue out of her mouth. There is a bilateral postural tremor of her arms with additional chorea and dystonic posturing. She has freezing of gait, mainly on turning, and postural reflexes loss.

25 Generalized Dystonia with Oromandibular Involvement and Self-mutilations: Lesch–Nyhan Syndrome

Roberto Erro and Kailash P. Bhatia

Clinical History and Investigations

This 19-year-old man with no family history had his first symptoms at age 9–10 months. He was noted to have developmental delay, along with frequent episodes of fever and abnormal posturing, mainly of his shoulders and the neck. He was first diagnosed with cerebral palsy, but a marked progression of his symptoms was noted thereafter. He developed abnormal posturing of his limbs, dysarthria, and dysphagia. Moreover, he had a number of seizures and further developed minor self-harm behaviours. He was noted to bite his lips and grind his teeth, causing extreme discomfort so that these were removed. He has also had episodes of renal colic with known renal stones. Following this, a diagnostic re-evaluation was performed, which led to the final diagnosis of Lesch–Nyhan syndrome. He was in fact found to have urinary urate-to-creatinine ratio greater than 2, indicating uric acid overproduction and suggesting the diagnosis. HPRT enzyme activity was measured in cultured fibroblasts and found to be less than 1.5 per cent, thus confirming a diagnosis of Lesch–Nyhan syndrome.

Examination

At the age of 19 years (see Video 25.1), he was alert and understood and followed basic commands. There was generalized dystonia, most prominently on the oromandibular and cervical region, with mouth-opening dystonia and protrusion of a hypertrophic tongue as well as torticollis to the left with a retrocollic component. He also had dystonic posturing of his hands and eversion of his feet. Intermittently, he had episodes where his eyes would shoot up to one side. These episodes last for several seconds, during which he could not respond in his usual fashion, suggestive of oculogyric crises. Ambulation was impossible.

Remarks

Lesch–Nyhan syndrome is an X-linked disorder caused by deficiency of the HPRT enzyme, which catalyzes the conversion of hypoxanthine to inosine monophosphate (inosinic acid) and guanine to guanine monophosphate (guanylic acid) in the presence of phosphoribosylpyrophosphate, and thus leading to uric acid overproduction.

Affected patients typically have a normal prenatal and perinatal course, but become symptomatic by the first year of life, with hypotonia and delayed motor skills usually evident by age 3–6 months. Children with Lesch–Nyhan syndrome fail to reach normal milestones such as sitting, crawling, and walking. Within the first few years of life, abnormal involuntary movements develop, and the characteristic feature is severe action dystonia, with prominent oromandibular and bulbar involvement. Patients can also develop choreoathetosis, opisthotonos, and sometimes ballismus. Additional symptoms include spasticity, hyperreflexia, and extensor plantar reflexes. The neurologic picture can resemble the athetoid variant of CP and, in fact, many affected children are initially misdiagnosed as having CP. The motor disability is so severe that virtually all affected subjects with the classic Lesch–Nyhan syndrome never walk and are highly dependent for their activities of daily life. Cognition is usually impaired and patients have additional and attentional problems and behavioural disturbances. Almost all affected individuals eventually develop persistent self-injurious behaviours, including biting of the fingers, hands, lips, and cheeks, a feature considered a hallmark of the disease, as well as head banging and injuries to the limbs. Other compulsive behaviours may include aggressiveness, vomiting, spitting, and coprolalia.

Lesch–Nyhan syndrome suspicion is very high when the three key elements of uric acid overproduction (with nephrolithiasis and/or hematuria), neurologic dysfunction, and behavioural disturbances with self-injuries are present. It should be noted, however, that a similar phenotype with self-injuries can occur in Chorea-acanthocytosis (cf. Case 36), even though the onset of the latter is classically later and patients most common present indeed with chorea rather than with generalized dystonia. Also, self-injurious behaviours can be present in other conditions such as Rett's syndrome, Tourette's, autism, and other psychiatric conditions.

Urinary urate-to-creatinine ratio higher than 2, 24-hour urate excretion of more than 20 mg/kg, and hyperuricemia (>8 mg/dL) are characteristic but not diagnostic. The diagnosis instead relies on HPRT enzyme assay or on molecular testing of the *HPRT1* gene.

The overproduction of uric acid must be controlled with allopurinol to reduce the risk for nephrolithiasis, urate nephropathy, gouty arthritis, and tophi. The dose of allopurinol is adjusted to maintain the uric acid within normal limits. However, control of serum concentration of uric acid has no effect on the development and progression behavioural and neurologic symptoms.

If management of symptoms is effective, most individuals survive into the second or third decade of life. Death is often due to respiratory abnormalities and aspiration pneumonia. Atlantoaxial subluxation due to forcible opisthotonos has been rarely reported as a cause of sudden death.

Suggested Readings

Jinnah HA, Friedmann T. Lesch–Nyhan disease and its variants. In: Valle D, Beaudet AL, Vogelstein B, et al., eds. *The Online Metabolic and Molecular Bases of Inherited Disease (OMMBID)*. 2015. New York: McGraw-Hill. Chap. 107.

Robey KL, Reck JF, Giacomini KD, Barabas G, Eddey GE. Modes and patterns of self-mutilation in persons with Lesch–Nyhan disease. *Dev Med Child Neurol.* 2003;45:167–71.

Schretlen DJ, Ward J, Meyer SM, et al. Behavioral aspects of Lesch–Nyhan disease and its variants. *Dev Med Child Neurol.* 2005;47:673–7.

 Video 25.1

This patient has generalized dystonia with prominent oromandibular involvement and tongue protrusion. The video also shows one episode of neck turning and eye version, suggestive of an oculogyric crisis. Both feet are everted, and an extensor plantar response of the left foot is shown. He has a patch of scopolamine for excessive drooling.

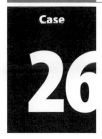

Dystonia Complicated by Pyramidal Signs, Parkinsonism, and Cognitive Impairment: HSP11

Roberto Erro, Maria Stamelou, and Kailash P. Bhatia

Clinical History

This 27-year-old man from a consanguineous family had normal birth and motor milestones. He started having postural and writing tremor by the age of 14. He then developed walking difficulties with imbalance, speech and swallowing issues, and slowness. His gait became progressively stiff and he had a few falls. His parents further reported that he was developing progressive memory difficulties and became apathetic. After an initial worsening over the first 6 or 7 years, the clinical picture was reported to be fairly stable.

Examination

On examination, he presented with facial hypomimia and up-gaze skew deviation with slowed upward eye movements. He had laryngeal dystonia. There was abnormal posturing of his hand and he had writing tremor with micrographia. There was also bilateral bradykinesia on repetitive movements and axial rigidity. His gait was markedly stiff, with spasticity and additional dystonic elements. Deep tendon reflexes were brisk and polyphasic bilaterally in the lower limbs, and he had bilateral ankle clonus. The remaining neurological examination was normal.

General Remarks

Although the symptoms at onset were those of postural and writing tremor, this patient developed further symptoms during the course of his disease. His phenotype indeed encompassed a combination of extrapyramidal (dystonia and parkinsonism) and pyramidal symptoms, the latter being the most prominent at the time of the examination. In such cases, the differential diagnosis is very wide and includes rare genetic forms of parkinsonism (cf. Table 3.1) as well as NBIA syndromes (cf. Table 23.1). However, in these conditions pyramidal signs are not usually the main feature and complicated forms of HSP, which can in fact present

with additional extrapyramidal symptoms and cognitive issues, should also be considered.

Investigations and Diagnosis

Basic serum investigations, including copper and ceruloplasmin, were normal. An MRI brain scan revealed marked supratentorial volume loss with an extremely thin corpus callosum (Figure 26.1). A DaT-Scan showed decreased bilateral putaminal and caudate uptake. Genetic testing of the *spatacsin* gene reveled a 2bp deletion (c.733_734delAT), thus leading to a diagnosis of HSP11.

Special Remarks

HSP11 (or SPG11) is one of the autosomal recessive complicated forms of HSP, with onset during childhood or puberty, and characteristically associated with a thin corpus callosum on brain imaging. HSP11 accounts for up to 14 per cent of all complicated forms of HSP, but up to 42 per cent of patients with thin corpus callosum. It classically presents with a slowly progressive spastic paraparesis associated with moderate to severe mental impairment, and a progressive thinning of the corpus callosum. Additional symptoms, including upper extremity weakness, peripheral neuropathy, dysarthria, cerebellar ataxia, extrapyramidal signs, epileptic seizures, and bladder dysfunction, have been variably described, and account for a marked variability of the clinical picture, even within the same families. Ophthalmological symptoms, including macular degeneration, strabismus, or cataract, and eye movement abnormalities have also been reported. As far as extrapyramidal signs are concerned, these can encompass dystonia, tremor, and parkinsonism, with the additional evidence of an abnormal DaT-Scan. Tremor, as in our case, has been reported as the initial symptom in a few other patients. In fact, after the identification of the gene, unusual phenotypes are increasingly being recognized. Given the possible variability in the clinical

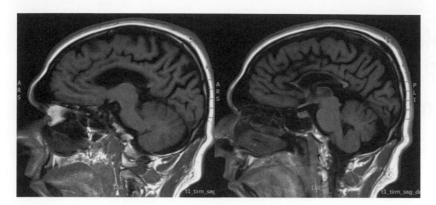

Figure 26.1 Sagittal MRI T1-sequences showing supratentorial atrophy with extremely thin corpus callosum.

presentation, the presence of marked pyramidal sings in the lower limbs with the evidence of a thin corpus callosum on the MRI should prompt the genetic testing of the *spatacsin* gene.

Suggested Readings

Abdel Aleem A, Abu-Shahba N, Swistun D, et al. Expanding the clinical spectrum of SPG11 gene mutations in recessive hereditary spastic paraplegia with thin corpus callosum. *Eur J Med Genet*. 2011;54:82–5.

Paisán-Ruiz C, Guevara R, Federoff M, et al. Early-onset L-dopa-responsive parkinsonism with pyramidal signs due to ATP13A2, PLA2G6, FBXO7 and spatacsin mutations. *Mov Disord*. 2010;25:1791–800.

Schneider SA, Mummery CJ, Mehrabian M, Houlden H, Bain PG. SPG11 presenting with tremor. *Tremor Other Hyperkinet Mov (N Y)*. 2012;2. pii: tre-02-104-666-1.

27

H-ABC Syndrome

Roberto Erro and Kailash P. Bhatia

Clinical History

A 30-year-old woman with no family history started having several falls by age 2, which were attributed to unsteadiness and clumsiness. Over the following 4–5 years she was further noted to have writing difficulties, an action tremor of her right hand, and speech problems, her voice appearing 'whispering' with increased tension on phonation. Examination at the age of 10 years showed a generalized dystonic syndrome, mainly involving her right arm but also affecting her feet on walking and her vocal cords. Her symptoms were progressive and progressively affected her walking, so that by age 19 years, she required a wheelchair for long distances. Her voice dysfunction progressed and she became aphonic by the age of 24.

Examination

On examination (see Video 27.1), it was revealed that she could not speak and protrude her tongue. Ocular movements were normal, but she had to blink to initiate saccades. There was a generalized dystonia with prominent oromandubular involvement and facial grimacing. There was mild ataxia on finger–nose test, with terminal tremor bilaterally. She had difficulties in performing repetitive movements particularly with her right hand. Unaided walking was impossible. She had pyramidal signs, including weakness in the upper limbs and bilateral extensor plantar reflex. The remaining neurological examination was normal.

General Remarks

The combination of generalized dystonia with a 'whispering' voice could raise the suspicion of 'hereditary whispering dysphonia' (also known as DYT4, cf. Table 16.1). However, in DYT4, pyramidal and cerebellar signs are not classically described and, in fact, this complex phenotype, along with the marked progression over time, suggests a heredodegenerative or metabolic disorder (cf. Table 22.1). A broad diagnostic work should be performed accordingly.

Investigations and Diagnosis

Serum and urine investigations, including copper and ceruloplasmin, very-long fatty acid chain, white cell enzymes, and organic acids, were all normal. An MRI brain scan revealed T2 weighted supratentorial diffuse hypomyelination and atrophy of basal ganglia (putaminal), with loss of cerebellar volume (Figure 27.1), suggesting the diagnosis of H-ABC syndrome. Genetic analysis of the *TUBB4A* gene showed that she carried the c.941C>T mutation in exon 4, thus confirming the diagnosis.

Special Remarks

H-ABC syndrome is a rare disorder due to *TUBB4A* mutations that, as the name suggests, is defined by a specific MRI pattern, featuring hypomyelination with atrophy of the basal ganglia and cerebellum. This specific radiological pattern clearly differentiates H-ABC from other genetically defined hypomyelinating disorders. It should, however, be noted that since the discovery of *TUBB4A* as causative for this syndrome, several neuroradiological patterns have been associated with H-ABC, some of which include isolated hypomyelination with no atrophy of both basal ganglia and cerebellum.

Clinically, patients show a phenotypic continuum with onset ranging from neonatal to childhood, normal to delayed early development, and slow to more rapid neurological deterioration, which is, however, invariably noted in all cases and usually lead to wheelchair dependence within the first two decades. Neurological features consist of dystonia with prominent oromandibular involvement, with additional spasticity and ataxia, while cognitive deficits and epilepsy are only rarely observed.

Interestingly, *TUBB4A* mutations have been described as causative for a seemingly different

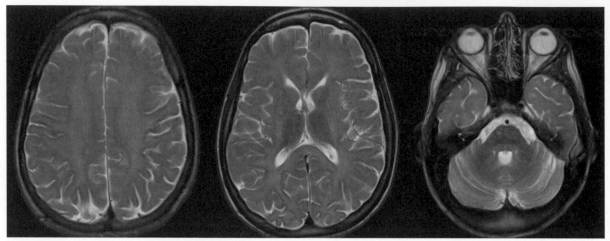

Figure 27.1 Axial MRI T1-sequences showing, left to right, diffuse supratentorial hypomyelination, putaminal atrophy, with relative preservation of the cerebrum.

disorder, DYT4 'hereditary whispering dysphonia', which was first described in a large Australian kindred. DYT4 is characterized by dysphonia (clinically of the 'whispering' type), severe generalized dystonia, and an unusual 'hobby horse' gait present in some of the affected cases. Although patients with DYT4 have been reported to have normal brain imaging, there are a number of clinical similarities between DYT4 and H-ABC patients, suggesting a continuous clinical and radiological spectrum associated with *TUBB4A* mutations.

Suggested Readings

Erro R, Hersheson J, Ganos C, et al. H-ABC syndrome and DYT4: variable expressivity or pleiotropy of TUBB4 mutations? *Mov Disord*. 2015;30:828–33.

Hamilton EM, Polder E, Vanderver A, et al. Hypomyelination with atrophy of the basal ganglia and cerebellum: further delineation of the phenotype and genotype-phenotype correlation. *Brain*. 2014;137:1921–30.

van der Knaap MS, Naidu S, Pouwels PJ, et al. New syndrome characterized by hypomyelination with atrophy of the basal ganglia and cerebellum. *AJNR Am J Neuroradiol*. 2002;23:1466–74.

 Video 27.1

There is generalized dystonia with prominent oromandubular involvement and facial grimacing. She is aphonic and cannot protrude her tongue. There is mild ataxia on finger–nose test and a terminal tremor bilaterally. She has difficulties in performing repetitive movements particularly with her right hand. Unaided walking is impossible. Bilateral extensor plantar reflex is shown.

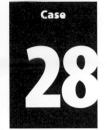

Tardive Dystonic Opisthotonus

Roberto Erro and Kailash P. Bhatia

Clinical History

A 63-year-old man with a long-standing history of major depression presented to our department for the appearance of involuntary movements mainly affecting his neck and trunk, which would abnormally spasm in hyper-extension, further causing pain. Such involuntary movements had begun approximately 2 years earlier and worsened over time, involving to a much lesser extent, his upper limbs, particularly the right one. Furthermore, on specific questioning, he reported that he was treated for many years with a combination of drugs, including typical antipsychotic.

Examination, Investigations, and Diagnosis

On examination (see Video 28.1), he showed marked retrocollis and dystonic opisthotonus at rest with additional facial grimaces. On walking, he had to hold his head with his left arm to avoid loosing his balance, but the abnormal posture of his trunk can still be seen. There are dystonic movements in his right arm. The remaining neurological examination was unremarkable. Standard blood investigations and a brain MRI turned out to be normal. Given the clinical picture, and on the basis of the long-term exposure to typical antipsychotic drugs, he was eventually diagnosed with tardive dystonia.

Remarks

The differential diagnosis of dystonic opisthotonus includes mainly secondary dystonias, while it is infrequent in primary dystonia. Opisthotonus have been described in neurometabolic disorders, including glutaric aciduria type 1, maple syrup urine disease, Lesch–Nyhan (cf. Table 22.1), and dopa-responsive dystonias. The very early age at onset and the association with other clinical features such as delayed motor milestones, truncal hypotonia, and encephalopathic crisis are helpful clues to suspect a neurometabolic disease. None of these conditions applies here and, pragmatically, there is only one disorder, namely tardive dystonia, which should be considered here, since as stated earlier, such a phenotype is very uncommon in primary dystonia. Retrocollis has been classically described in tardive dystonia caused by use of dopamine receptor antagonists. In fact, up to 50 per cent of patients with tardive dystonia have retrocollis, and about half of these also have extensor truncal dystonia, which worsens during movement, especially walking. Perioral dyskinesias and respiratory involvement, such as frequent grunting noises and irregular respiratory patterns, typical of tardive dyskinesias, can also occur. In summary, tardive dystonia can develop anytime after exposure to dopamine receptor blocking drugs, without predilection to any particular age group or sex. Patients can develop tardive dystonia even after relatively short duration of exposure to dopamine antagonists, in some cases after a few weeks. In theory, withdrawal of the offending medication should result in an improvement of the dystonia. However, clinical improvement occurs in only about half of the cases. Anticholinergic drugs or botulinum toxin injections can be somewhat helpful for tardive dystonia, but tetrabenazine seems to be the most effective drug in controlling tardive dyskinesias, with more than 50 per cent response rate. Pallidal DBS is highly effective for tardive dystonia and dyskinesias with improvement rates as good as primary dystonia.

Suggested Readings

Kang UJ, Burke RE, Fahn S. Natural history and treatment of tardive dystonia. *Mov Disord*. 1986;1:193–208.

Molho ES, Feustel PJ, Factor SA. Clinical comparison of tardive and idiopathic cervical dystonia. *Mov Disord*. 1998;13:486–9.

Video 28.1

There is a severe retrocollis as well as a mild extensor trunk dystonia. This patient has to hold his head tight to not lose his balance when walking.

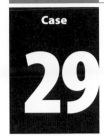

Delayed Onset Dystonia after Lightning Strike

Roberto Erro and Kailash P. Bhatia

Clinical History

This 25-year-old woman started having involuntary movements with abnormal posturing following an accident when she was 15. She was walking in a park in London and talking on her mobile phone during a violent thunderstorm. Unfortunately, she was struck by lightning that first hit her phone to eventually exit through her left foot (Figure 29.1A and B). She collapsed and has been in asystolic arrest for about 7 minutes. When a helicopter ambulance arrived, she was found lying on the floor, with her left arm being held rigidly upwards and a burnt-out mobile phone clutched in her hand. There was no cardiac activity and she was therefore given resuscitation and adrenaline, with success. Initial CT scan apparently showed some areas of increased signal with edema and there were said to be some hypoxic ischemic changes. She had been under the care of the pediatricians and slowly became conscious, making a good recovery despite having significant memory recall difficulties as to her accident. She afterwards (some months later) started having some left foot abnormal posturing, which deteriorated over the years and spread to other body districts and was hence referred to us as to further possible management.

Examination

On examination, it was observed that she had a hypomimic face and was almost anarthric. She had a generalized dystonia, which was more severe in her lower limbs. She could not walk unaided, tending to extend her trunk backwards both when attempting to stand and to sit. Her postural reflexes tested abnormal. Moreover, she was quite slow on finger tapping. The remaining neurological examination was unremarkable.

Investigations

A brain MRI scan showed mineralization in the posterior part of the putamen bilaterally (Figure 29.1C). A DaT-Scan was proven to be abnormal, with decreased binding in both putamen and relative sparing of the caudate nuclei.

Remarks

According to data from the National Oceanic and Atmospheric Administration, in the years from 1959 to 1994, lightning was responsible for over 3,000 deaths and nearly 10,000 casualties, but actual numbers might be even higher since a large proportion of lightning strikes are unreported. Cardiac arrest is the main and most common cause of death following lightning strikes. However, for those who survive, the most devastating complications are undoubtedly neurologic. Although CNS damage following lightning and electrical injuries has been largely documented in the literature, documentation of movement disorders after lightning strikes is rather sparse.

Described in general, neurological manifestations following lightning injuries can be grouped according to their timing of appearance and putative pathophysiology into four categories: *immediate and transient symptoms*, including loss of consciousness, amnesia, confusion, headache, paresthesia, and weakness; *immediate and prolonged or permanent symptoms*, which result from post hypoxic-ischemic encephalopathy, and intracranial hemorrhages and/or ischemia; *lightning-linked secondary trauma from falls or blast*; and *delayed and progressive neurologic syndromes*. The latter group includes reports of motor neuron disease and movement disorders following lightning strikes by days to months to years. This seemed the case in our patient, who first developed abnormal posturing of her left foot a few months after her accident. Moreover, her symptoms were progressive over time, despite an initial good recovery from the acute phase.

The cause–effect relationship between lightning and subsequent delayed complications is, however, not entirely clear. Different mechanisms (either central or peripheral) have been suggested to account for the movement disorders observed in these patients

Table 29.1 Possible Mechanisms for Movement Disorders Induced by Lightning or Electrical Injury

Movement Disorder	Central Mechanisms	Peripheral Mechanisms
Parkinsonism	- Basal ganglia ischemia - Cerebral anoxia	None known
Dystonia	- Basal ganglia ischemia - Cerebral anoxia	Associated with reflex sympathetic dystrophy (questioned)
Choreo-athesosis	- Basal ganglia ischemia - Cerebral anoxia	Proprioceptive tract damage (pseudoathetosis)
Myoclonus	- Basal ganglia ischemia - Cerebral anoxia	Spinal cord lesion (segmental myoclonus)
Tremor	Cerebellar outflow tract ischemia	None known

Source: Modified from O'Brien, 1995.

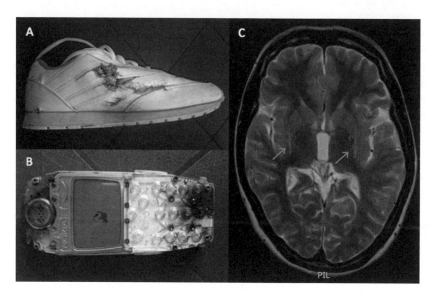

Figure 29.1 (A) Left shoe with a hole, through which the lightning exited; (B) Burnt-out mobile phone that our patient was holding when struck by the lightning; (C) Axial T2-sequence showing bilateral hyperintensity (mineralization) in the posterior putamen (arrows). A black and white version of this figure will appear in some formats. For the colour version, please refer to the plate section.

(Table 29.1). Central mechanisms are supposed to act through anoxia and/or ischemia. Yet, such mechanisms would not entirely explain why symptoms develop after a certain time from the injury or why they are progressive. Delayed movements disorders following post-hypoxic encephalopathy from other types of injuries have also been reported, remarking the selective vulnerability of the basal ganglia in such circumstances.

Notably, in our case there was evidence of an abnormal DaT-Scan (performed because of the further appearance of parkinsonian features), in the absence of midbrain lesions on MRI. It is generally assumed that post-synaptic lesions (as in this case, whose MRI showed mineralization of the posterior putamen bilaterally) do not produce abnormal DaT-Scan, even though this possibility cannot be entirely ruled out. Thus, such an intriguing evidence might suggest that the progressive dysfunction of basal ganglia outflow after hypoxia could over the long term determine degeneration of the presynaptic terminals, through some sort of 'dying-back' mechanism. Yet, such hypothesis remains entirely speculative and warrants further investigation.

Suggested Readings

Burke RE, Fahn S, Gold AP. Delayed-onset dystonia in patients with 'static' encephalopathy. *J Neurol Neurosurg Psychiatry*. 1980;43(9):789–97.

Cherington M. Neurologic manifestations of lightning strikes. *Neurology*. 2003;60(2):182–5.

O'Brien CF. Involuntary movement disorders following lightning and electrical injuries. *Semin Neurol*. 1995;15(3):263–7.

Case

30

Gilles de la Tourette Syndrome

Christos Ganos

History

A 38-year-old gentleman, who had normal early development, manifested excess and intrusive movements at the age of 6. They consisted of simple, localized repetitive motor behaviours, such as eye blinking, eye rolling, head turning but also more complex motor phenomena such as sudden turning or kneeling down. At the same period he also vocalized loudly (e.g. 'ah', 'pah') or intermittently made sounds resembling barking. These movements/phonations persisted throughout the ensuing years, albeit waxing and waning in frequency and intensity. They were preceded by an increasing and unpleasant sensation that the patient described as tension, a need to move, or tightness around his neck that briefly ceased upon movement execution or loud vocalization. The patient also had difficulties concentrating for longer periods of time and had, therefore, problems in completing his school tasks. By the age of 10, he was evaluated by several medical doctors and he was eventually diagnosed with an unspecified allergic reaction and was forbidden from eating sweets. At the age of 12, following a subsequent evaluation at the child medicine department of a university clinic, the diagnosis of GTS was given. During that same period the patient also developed obsessions and compulsions, such as the need to fastidiously order his books and toys, to repetitively touch certain items three times, to pause while climbing stairs at every fourth step, and to unsuccessfully pursue counting to 1,000 without permitting tics to occur. Two brief treatment attempts with haloperidol at the age of 14 and tiapride one year later were both discontinued due to side effects, such as severe sedation, withdrawal, and depression. Thereafter, the patient did not wish to attempt any further medication, and it was only upon completing his basic education that he sought further medical help and was then, aged 20, treated with pimozide (4 mg/day). This resulted in a sustained overall improvement of his tics associated with a reduction of the preceding unpleasant sensations. With regard to his reduced concentration ability and his OCB, he felt that they were not a cause of distress nor a reason to take further medications. Worth noting, from the age of 24 and to the present time, he also developed the need to perform obscene, but void of intent, movements, or expressions, such as showing the middle finger while speaking or repetitively and suddenly uttering swearwords while speaking. A severe jaw-opening tic with lateral deviation of the mandible, which he developed at the age of 34 and which had caused significant local pain was successfully treated with local botulinum toxin injections into his right lateral pterygoid muscle.

Examination

Neurological examination (Video 30.1) was unremarkable but for the presence of several simple and complex motor and phonic tics, including echo-, pali-, and copro-phenomena.

Remarks

Tic disorders are among the most common hyperkinesias with an estimated prevalence of up to 0.8 per cent in children. Tic disorders are most frequently encountered as primary syndromes, notably in GTS. According to DSM-5, this diagnosis can be given in the presence of chronic (i.e. >12 months) and multiple motor and vocal (or phonic) tics, with onset before the age of 18 and in the absence of secondary causes. The patient presented here indeed fulfilled these diagnostic criteria. Crucially, the patient's early development was normal and there were not any further relevant medical history or neurological signs that would hint towards a secondary condition. The patient's tics showed the characteristic for primary tic disorders pattern of waxing and waning, as well as fluctuations in tic repertoire over time. The presence of typical echo- and paliphenomena, commonly encountered in primary tic disorders, further reinforced diagnostic certainty.

Moreover, the patient had persistent difficulties with concentration, albeit not prominent hyperactivity or impulsivity, and although no formal neuropsychiatric assessment was performed, it appears that he might have had symptoms of ADHD. In addition, around his early adolescence he developed OCB, for which, he did not, though, pursue any treatment. Both ADHD and OCB (as well as OCD) are common neuropsychiatric comorbidities within the GTS spectrum (up to 90 per cent of cases). Of note, ASD has also been associated with tics and GTS (cf. Case 33). It should be noted that clinicians should enquire for the presence of additional psychopathological behaviours, as for example self-injurious behaviour, anxiety and personality disorders, as well as depressive illness (lifetime risk of 10 per cent).

As to treatment, recognizing the correct diagnosis and communicating the neurological background, as well as the natural course of tics and GTS (psychoeducation), is of paramount importance. Only then and in the minority of cases, such as the one demonstrated here, where tics are sources of discomfort and/or pain, or interfere with the patient's social life leading to stigmatization (e.g. due to coprophenomena), are further treatment steps required. Pharmacological agents, including neuroleptics, tetrabenazine or alpha-2 adrenergic agonists, or botulinum toxin injections for particularly troubling tics, and non-pharmacological approaches, such as habit-reversal training, can all be employed tailored to the individual needs and goals of patients.

Suggested Readings

Ganos C, Martino D. Tics and Tourette syndrome. *Neurol Clin*. 2015;33:115–36.

Ganos C, Roessner V, Munchau A. The functional anatomy of Gilles de la Tourette syndrome. *Neurosci Biobehav Rev*. 2013;37:1050–62.

Ganos C, Martino D, and Pringsheim T. Tics in the pediatric population: pragmatic management. *Mov Disord Clin Pract*. 2016. doi:10.1002/mdc3.12428.

Jankovic J. Tourette syndrome. Phenomenology and classification of tics. *Neurol Clin*. 1997;15:267–75.

Robertson MM. A personal 35 year perspective on Gilles de la Tourette syndrome: prevalence, phenomenology, comorbidities, and coexistent psychopathologies. *The Lancet Psychiatry*. 2015;2:68–87.

Video 30.1

The patient is being filmed while alone in a room. Video demonstrates a repertoire of multiple simple and complex motor and phonic tics.

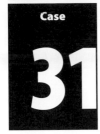

Case

31

Secondary Tic Disorders: HD

Christos Ganos and Kailash P. Bhatia

This 57-year-old gentleman, who had no relevant past medical record, presented with a 7-year history of abnormal excess movements. His first symptoms affected the legs and were described as twitching and fidgeting, manifesting particularly in the evening. His symptoms progressed to also involve the arms and face, and they became more constant throughout the day. He could completely stop the movements willingly, but only for brief moments, due to a rising unpleasant sensation of tightness/tension. Three years prior to current presentation, he was diagnosed with late onset tic disorder and had been treated with tetrabenazine, which led to a dramatic improvement of his motor symptoms. However, approximately two years later, he became severely depressed and also experienced a worsening of his movement disorder, with the new manifestation of vocalizations alongside more severe twitches and jerks of his body. Tetrabenazine was discontinued and subsequent medication trials with clonazepam, risperidone, and clonidine showed no clear benefit. The patient's father was reported to have mild excess movements, dysarthria, and poor balance. Further family history was unrevealing.

Examination

Clinical examination (Video 31.1) revealed marked oculomotor abnormalities, with gaze impersistence, and difficulty in initiating voluntary saccades with compensatory head thrust. He was unable to keep his tongue protruded for longer periods of time. There was no abnormality in examination of strength, reflexes, or somatosensation. He had an unusual gait with dystonic posturing affecting his right leg. His postural stability was good. There was no ataxia. With regard to the abnormal movements, there was a mixed hyperkinetic movement disorder dominated by motor and phonic tics, with elements of chorea and the aforementioned dystonia.

Investigations

Laboratory investigations, basic blood tests, creatine kinase levels – including acanthocytes and copper studies – a brain MRI scan, and repeated EEGs were all normal.

Diagnosis

Given the clinical presentation of a late onset tic disorder with chorea, dystonia, and neuropsychiatric manifestations (depression), as well as a possible positive autosomal-dominant family history, the diagnosis of HD was considered. Indeed, mutation analysis for expansions in the *IT15* gene revealed a pathologically expanded allele of 42 (± 2 repeats) repeats and a normal allele with 18 repeats, thereby confirming the clinical diagnosis.

Remarks

Despite difficulties in recognizing GTS in the past, the contemporary diagnosis of a primary tic disorder/GTS is, in most cases, straightforward. However, there are certain diagnostic caveats in discerning tics from other movement disorders. This case is a clear example of (secondary) tics as part of the clinical presentation of another condition. Here, a patient with no prior medical history, and no history of tic disorders in childhood, insidiously developed motor and phonic tics in his sixth life decade. Clearly, the onset age is much older than the transitional age of adolescent to adulthood, which is used as a cut off for primary tic disorders. Therefore, a secondary cause of tics was considered. Such causes comprise neurodevelopmental disorders, including (X-)chromosomal disorders, neurometabolic disorders, structural brain lesions, drug-induced tics, as well as tics associated with neurodegenerative syndromes. Given the absence of any relevant past medical history, including past pharmacological treatments, the normal brain MRI, the progressive course of the patients symptoms, and the possibly positive paternal family history, a neurodegenerative disorder was readily considered. Within this spectrum of disorders, given the patient's age at symptom onset, FTD, HD, ChAc, and NBIA, particularly neuroferritinopathy, should be considered. The mixed hyperkinetic movement disorder at the time of presentation, consisting of tics and chorea with some additional dystonia, in the absence of clear ataxia and clinical, as well as electrophysiological, signs of peripheral neuropathy hinted to the diagnosis of HD, which was, indeed, subsequently genetically confirmed.

Suggested Readings

Ganos C, Münchau A, Bhatia K. The semiology of tics, Tourette's and their associations. *Mov Disord Clin Pract* 2014;1:149–53.

Kurlan R. *Handbook of Tourette's syndrome and related tic and behavioral disorders.* 2005, 2nd ed. New York: Marcel Dekker.

Mejia NI, Jankovic J. Secondary tics and tourettism. *Rev Bras Psiquiatr.* 2005;27:11–17.

 Video 31.1

Patient gives brief description of his medical history. Video demonstrates multiple simple and complex motor tics, as well as prominent simple phonic tics and generalized chorea. He also appears restless (he had not been treated with neuroleptics). Hyperkinetic movements are only partially suppressible for a very brief period of time (< 5 seconds). There is no bradykinesia or upper limb ataxia. Gait appears stiff with clear dystonic posturing of the right leg.

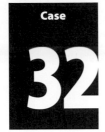

Multiple Hyperkinesias: Tics and Paroxysmal Kinesigenic Dyskinesia

Christos Ganos and Kailash P. Bhatia

This 19-year-old boy had a history of three seizures during the first 18 months of his life. He was subsequently diagnosed with ADHD at the age of 5 and, for that, he had been receiving methylphenidate for 5 years. Aged 7 he developed several motor and phonic tics, such as excessive eye blinking, eye rolling, frowning, tongue rolling, shoulder shrugging, sniffing, and grunting, and he was diagnosed with GTS. Although he did not suffer from severe obsessions/compulsions, he did, indeed, meticulously order his video games and repetitively check door locks. According to a neuropsychiatric evaluation at the age of 9, he was also diagnosed with ASD. There was a positive maternal family history for infantile seizures and migraine, as well as a report of a maternal cousin diagnosed with ASD.

Aged 17, he was referred to our department for the treatment of disruptive motor behaviours, which had first appeared around the age of 14 years and were diagnosed as complex tics. These behaviours appeared abruptly/episodic, lasted for less than a minute (usually < 30 seconds) and consisted of cramping and twisting of, predominantly, the right side of his body (Video 32.1A). There appeared to be a somatotopic distribution of the episodes, with the feet initially being affected, but spreading to involve the trunk, arms, and on occasion cranial muscles, particularly the jaw with inability to articulate. There was little phenomenological variability between episodes, which could, however, occur with different intensity between 5 and 100 times a day and were triggered by sudden movements or loud noises. Prior to their occurrence, they were briefly preceded by generalized tension or focal numbness of the calves. The patient, although fully conscious, had no control over these episodes but when able, he attempted to suppress their full expression by holding down the affected extremity. According to the patient, the two classes of excess movements – tics from young age and the aforementioned episodic movements that appeared in a latter age – clearly differed in that he experienced the latter to be completely involuntary.

Examination

Examination revealed the presence of simple and complex motor tics, echo- and paliphenomena, as well as simple phonic tics (Video 32.1B). Most of his tics could be inhibited on demand. No additional movements, in particular, no cramping or twisting were noted during examination, despite attempts to elicit such.

Investigations

Previous examinations (interictal EEG, brain MRI, acanthocytes, serum copper/ceruloplasmin, white cell enzymes) were normal.

Diagnosis and Remarks

Given the unusual character of the episodic movements from the age of 14, their duration and phenomenological invariability, as well as the presence of triggers, and the patient's report on their qualitative distinction from his pre-existing tics, the diagnosis of paroxysmal kinesigenic dyskinesia in addition to that of GTS and ADHD was considered. Indeed, the presence of infantile convulsions in the patient and his mother, as well as the positive maternal family history for migraine, supported this clinical diagnosis. Genetic analysis of the Proline-Rich Transmembrane Protein 2 (*PRRT2*) gene confirmed diagnosis; the patient was found to be a heterozygous carrier of the c.649dupC (p.R217P fs*8) mutation, which has been recognized as the most common causative mutation for familial paroxysmal kinesigenic dyskinesia. The patient was initially treated with 100 mg Carbamazepine, which led to an impressive cessation of his attacks, without having

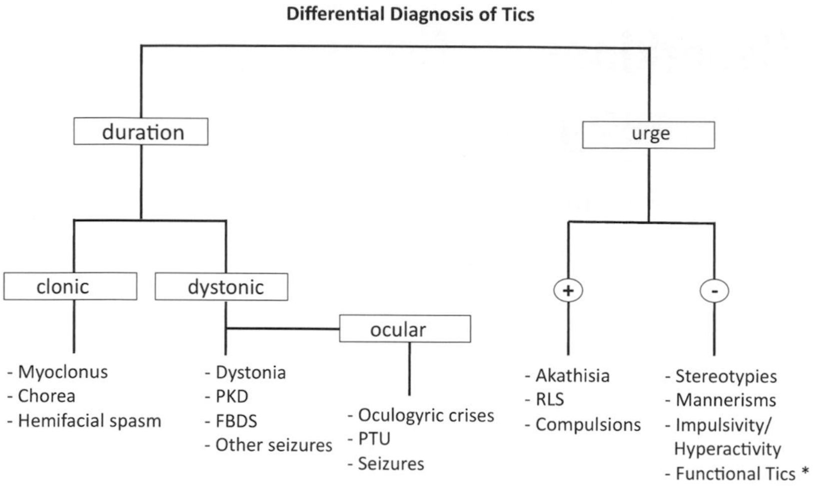

Differential Diagnosis of Tics

Figure 32.1 A clinical approach to the differential diagnosis of tics.

Source: Adapted from Ganos C, Münchau A, Bhatia K. The semiology of tics, Tourette's and their associations. *Mov Disord Clin Pract*. 2014;1:149–54.

(FBDS, facio-brachial dystonic seizures; PKD, paroxysmal kinesigenic dyskinesia; PTU, paroxysmal tonic upgaze; RLS, restless legs syndrome. A nonlocalized premonitory sensation may be reported.)

Table 32.1 Movement Disorders Other Than Tics Co-occurring in GTS

Primary	Dystonia
	PLM
	Stereotypies
Secondary	Dystonia
	Akathisia
	Chorea
	PKD*

Source: Adapted from Ganos C, Münchau A, Bhatia K. The semiology of tics, Tourette's and their associations. *Mov Disord Clin Pract*. 2014;1:149–53.
Abb.: *PLM = Periodic limb movements; PKD = Paroxysmal kinesigenic dyskinesia. The categorical division of primary versus secondary movement disorders refers to the possibility of the additional movement disorder being either part of the pathophysiological spectrum of GTS or a result of medication or a different medical condition. * = The pathophysiological relation between PKD and GTS currently remains unclear.*

any effect on his tics. Over the ensuing two years, as the patient still occasionally felt some tension or tightness around his calves, without, though, experiencing an attack, the dosage was increased to 300 mg a day with complete resolution of all symptoms.

Indeed tics (and GTS) have been reported to co-occur in patients with PKD. However, it is unclear, whether this association is co-incidental or has a shared pathophysiological background. Interestingly, PRRT2 interacts with the synaptosomal associated protein of 25 kD (SNAP-25), which has been associated with GTS. For example, the expression levels of SNAP-25 in peripheral blood correlated with tic severity of medication – naive GTS children and adolescents.

Obviously, GTS patients may also present with other additional movement disorders the recognition of which may have important implication for treatment. These most commonly include secondary movement disorders, as, for example, drug-related (i.e. neuroleptic-induced) movement disorders, such as acute akathisia or acute dystonic reactions. Tardive movement disorders may also occur in this context; however, there is no good systematic evidence for their presence in patients with GTS. Finally, the distinction between dystonia and (dystonic) tics can also pose diagnostic difficulties in some cases, and co-occurrence of tics and dystonia has been reported. Table 32.1 summarizes a list of additional movement disorders that may co-occur in GTS, and Figure 32.1 demonstrates a clinical approach in the differential diagnosis of tics.

Suggested Readings

Damasio J, Edwards MJ, Alonso-Canovas A, Schwingenschuh P, Kagi G, Bhatia KP. The clinical syndrome of primary tic disorder associated with dystonia: a large clinical series and a review of the literature. *Mov Disord*. 2011;26:679–84.

Erro R, Sheerin UM, Bhatia KP. Paroxysmal dyskinesias revisited: a review of 500 genetically proven cases and a new classification. *Mov Disord*. 2014;29:1108–16.

Erro R, Martino D, Ganos C, Damasio J, Batla A, Bhatia KP. Adult-onset primary dystonic tics: a different entity? *Mov Disord Clin Pract*. 2014;1:62–6.

Kompoliti K, Goetz CG. Hyperkinetic movement disorders misdiagnosed as tics in Gilles de la Tourette syndrome. *Mov Disord*. 1998;13:477–80.

Video 32.1

A: classic, short lasting (< 10 seconds in this segment) paroxysmal kinesigenic dyskinesia attack with generalized dystonic choreic-ballistic movements. B: hyperactive patient is being filmed while alone in room. Video demonstrates multiple simple and complex motor tics, as well as simple phonic tics.

33

Functional Tic Disorders

Christos Ganos

Shortly after a viral infection with flu-like symptoms, this 66-year-old man had a sudden episode of collapse with retained consciousness but complete inability to move over a period of several days. He was admitted into a hospital, where no cause was identified for this episode. An MRI of the brain and the spine during the episode were normal. Following hospital discharge, several less severe episodes occurred. About three months later, he developed very brief, sudden, and repetitive movements consisting of neck flexion, loud vocalizations, and arm flinging, while fully conscious (Video 33.1). There was no variability in these episodes, which occurred up to 20 times/hour if he was under pressure. There were no distinct premonitory sensations preceding the episodes, but a general feeling of pressure localized in the head and face throughout the day. The movements could not be interrupted or suppressed. There was no past neurological history and no report of tics during childhood, but a positive history of depression. The patient suffered from hypertension, gout, and wore bilateral hearing aids.

Examination

Neurological examination was normal but for occasional sudden episodes of neck flexion, loud vocalizations, and arm elevation (see Video 33.1).

Investigations

Laboratory examinations, including basic blood tests, creatine kinase levels, ASA titres, auto-antibodies in serum and CSF, repeated brain and spine MRI, electrophysiological assessments (nerve conduction studies, EMG, motor-evoked potentials, EEG during episodes) were all normal or unrevealing.

Diagnosis and Remarks

Upon exclusion of secondary causes of tic disorders and given the patient's sudden onset of symptoms, the atypical age of onset, the phenomenological invariability of

the episodes, the lack of a clear premonitory urge, and the inability to suppress the involuntary movements, the diagnosis of a functional tic disorder was given. The patient was subsequently referred to neuropsychiatry for further evaluation and treatment.

Among the different hyperkinetic movement disorders, the distinction of functional tic-like movements (or for simplicity functional tics) from organic tics can be particularly challenging. Irrespective of their origin, be it organic or functional, tics (and tic-like movements) resemble voluntary actions, they may be preceded by premotor potentials and are influenced by attention. Recently, however, certain clinical characteristics have been identified, which could aid discerning one type of movement from the other. First, age of symptom onset is crucial. According to DSM-5, primary tic disorders (with the exception of 'tic disorder not otherwise specified') have an onset prior to age 18, and in fact primary tics emerging at an atypical older age (>18 years) are exceptionally rare. Hence, the following possibilities should be primarily considered for a patient presenting with a tic disorder with onset in adulthood: (1) Patients become aware of their tics in adulthood, despite their presence from childhood; (2) Patients have a secondary tic disorder; and (3) Patients have a functional tic disorder. Second, the onset of organic tics is, particularly for primary tics, insidious. On the contrary, as also for other functional movement disorders, functional tics usually have an abrupt onset and may be associated with a physical or psychological precipitating event. Third, functional tics are rarely preceded by localized premonitory sensations/urges. Conversely, patients with organic tic disorders, particularly adults, commonly report the presence of premonitory sensations/urges, which in fact follow a similar distribution pattern (intensity and frequency) to that of tics. It is worth noting that although organic tics do show a somatotopic, rostro-caudal pattern of spatial distribution with the face being the most commonly affected area, this appears to differ in patients with functional tic disorders, where tic distribution is rather non-systematic. Fourth, most tics of organic origin can be voluntarily suppressed to some extent, whereas functional tics, as in the afore-mentioned case, usually cannot be subjected to the same amount of voluntary inhibitory control. Fifth, response of functional tics to anti-tic medication is disappointing. Sixth, patients with functional tics may present additional functional neurological symptoms, which might further aid diagnostic distinction. Finally, the neuropsychiatric profiles of patients with organic and functional tic disorders differ. Psychiatric condi-tions, such as ADHD and/or OCB/OCD are very com-mon in patients with organic tic disorders, but not in patients with functional tic disorders. However, anx-iety disorder and depression may be encountered in either group of patients.

Suggested Readings

Demartini B, Ricciardi L, Parees I, et al. A positive diagnosis of functional (psychogenic) tics. *Eur J Neurol.* 2015. 22:527–e36.

Dooley JM, Stokes A, Gordon KE. Pseudo-tics in Tourette's syndrome. *J Child Neurol.* 1994;9:50–1.

Ganos C, Edwards MJ, Müller-Vahl K. 'I swear it is Tourette's!': On functional coprolalia and other tic-like vocalizations. *Psychiatry Res.* 2016. doi: 10.1016/j.psychres.2016.10.021.

Eng-King T. Psychogenic tics: diagnostic value of the placebo test. *J Child Neurol.* 2004;19:976–7.

Kurlan R, Deeley C, Como PG. Psychogenic movement disorders (pseudo-tics) in a patient with Tourette's syndrome. *J Neuropsychiatry Clin Neurosci* 1992;4:347–8.

 Video 33.1

Brief, sudden, repetitive, and phenomenologically in-variable movements consisting of neck flexion, loud vocalizations, and arm flinging, while fully conscious. In one of these episodes the patient describes his awareness of a building pressure/pain in his head prior to the episode.

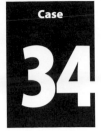

Chorea and Cognitive Difficulty: HD

Roberto Erro, Maria Stamelou and Kailash P. Bhatia

Clinical History

This 67-year-old man with no family history was referred for a 3-year history of involuntary movements and memory difficulties. He mentioned that he first noted twitching and fidgeting of his fingers and involuntary facial movements. He also reported that he had low mood and some memory difficulty.

Examination

On examination (see Video 34.1), he had involuntary movement mostly affecting his face. He had excessive blinking and involuntary movements of his upper face and perioral as well as choreic movements of his fingers and toes, most evident with distraction. He also had difficulty defixating, using a blink to initiate saccades. The remaining neurological examination was unremarkable.

General Remarks

Given the phenotype of chorea with onset in adulthood and the additional presence of mood and cognitive complaints, the clinical picture would be consistent with HD, even in the absence of a family history. The difficulty in initiating saccadic ocular movement would also fit with a diagnosis of HD. However, the differential diagnosis of HD is wide. In fact, other genetic conditions (Table 34.1) as well as acquired conditions such as polycythaemia rubra vera, systemic lupus erythematosis, and antiphospholipid syndrome can present with a similar phenotype. The diagnostic work-up should be pursued accordingly.

Investigations and Diagnosis

Biochemical investigations were all normal. A brain MRI revealed a marked volume reduction of the caudate bilaterally with additional frontal atrophy (cf. Figure 14.1). A genetic screening revealed that he carried 41 CAG repeats in the *IT15* gene, thus confirming the diagnosis of HD.

Special Remarks

HD is an autosomal dominant disorder caused by a CAG repeat expansion in exon 1 of the huntingtin gene (*HTT*, also known as *IT15*). There is a correlation between number of repeats and age at onset, and in successive generations onset tends to develop earlier in life (so-called genetic anticipation), particularly when inherited from the father.

The motor phenotype in HD is mainly characterized by chorea, but can encompass dystonia, parkinsonism, and rarely tics (cf. Case 31), with onset in midlife. However, the phenotype can be dominated by parkinsonism, especially in early onset (Westphal variant, cf. Case 14). Often, HD patients also demonstrate abnormal facial expression, gaze impersistence, impaired saccadic eye movements, with anti-saccadic movement almost invariably impaired, at least in the advanced stage of the disease. As far as the disease progresses, there is increasing postural instability and dysarthria as well as swallowing difficulties. Early in the course of the disease, personality changes or major psychiatric disorders (depression, anxiety, and suicidal thoughts) occur and often precede the onset of involuntary movements. Similarly, cognition (especially executive functions but later also memory function) is progressively affected.

There is no efficacious treatment for HD, with tetrabenazine being the most helpful medication for controlling the movement disorders. It has to be reminded, however, that it can exacerbate depression and, therefore, an adequate balance between the benefit and possible side effects needs to be achieved in individual cases.

Table 34.1 Summary of Genetic Disorders That Can Often Present with Adult Onset Chorea*

Condition	Gene	Pattern of inheritance	Age at onset	Clinical characteristics
HD	*IT5/HTT*	AD	Midlife (depends on the size of triplet expansion)	Chorea, personality changes, dementia
HDL1	*PRNP*	AD	20–40 years	HD phenocopy, prominent psychiatric features
HDL2	*JPH3*	AD	25–45 years	HD phenocopy or parkinsonism. Most frequent in black South Africans
HDL4 (SCA17)	TBP	AD	25–40 years	Ataxia, HD phenocopy
DRPLA	*ATN1*	AD	<20 years >40 years	PME Ataxia, chorea, dementia
Neuroferritinopathy	*FTL*	AD	40 years	Chorea, dystonia, oromandibular involvement, parkinsonism, dysarthria
–	*C9orf72*	AD	Variable (it ranges from the 2nd to the 8th decade)	Movement disorders, dementia, motor-neuron disease
Chorea-acanthocytosis	*VPS13A*	AR	30–40 years	Chorea, oromandibular dystonia, self-mutilations, seizures, myopathy, neuropathy
McLeod syndrome	*XK*	X-linked	50 years	Chorea, oromandibular dystonia, self-mutilations, seizures, myopathy, neuropathy, cardiomyopathy
–	*RNF216*	AR	30–40 years	Chorea, behavioural and cognitive disturbances, ataxia, pyramidal signs

* Note that occasionally SCA1, SCA2, SCA3, late onset Friedreich's Ataxia, and WD can present with chorea.

Suggested Readings

Gövert F, Schneider SA. Huntington's disease and Huntington's disease-like syndromes: an overview. *Curr Opin Neurol.* 2013;26:420–7.

Martino D, Stamelou M, Bhatia KP. The differential diagnosis of Huntington's disease-like syndromes: 'red flags' for the clinician. *J Neurol Neurosurg Psychiatry.* 2013;84(6):650–6.

Ross CA, Aylward EH, Wild EJ, et al. Huntington disease: natural history, biomarkers and prospects for therapeutics. *Nat Rev Neurol.* 2014;10:204–16.

Video 34.1

This patient has difficulties initiating saccades and has to blink to defixate. Moreover, there are choreic movements affecting his face and upper limbs.

Case

35

Generalized Chorea with Oromandibular Involvement and Tongue Biting: Chorea-acanthocytosis

Roberto Erro, Maria Stamelou, and Kailash P. Bhatia

Clinical History

This 40-year-old right-handed man with no known family history of any neurological conditions came to us due to development of involuntary movements. Around 8 years before, he first found himself to be not interested anymore in his job and social relationships and was diagnosed with depression and treated with fluoxetine, with a partial improvement. About 2 years later, he started to get involuntary movements around his mouth and tongue and had difficulty with his speech. His condition was progressive over time and his involuntary movements spread to his arms. In addition, he started having unsteadiness and a few falls occurred. He further developed eating difficulties with tongue biting. Moreover, his psychiatric symptoms got worse and he was also found to have some self-injury behaviors. Aged 39, he presented with his first generalized tonic-clonic seizure and developed progressive loss of bladder control.

Examination

On examination (see Video 35.1), he had generalized chorea. There was prominent orobulbar involvement with marked dysarthria and swallowing difficulties. Moreover, there was severe bruxism culminating in tongue biting and damage of his teeth. His gait was very unstable and lurching. The remaining neurological examination was unremarkable, apart from hypoactive deep tendon reflexes in his lower limbs.

General Remarks

Although the combination of chorea with psychiatric disturbances would first point towards a suspicion of HD (despite the absence of a positive family history), there are in this case other clinical clues suggesting an alternative diagnosis. A list of genetic disorders to consider in the differential diagnosis of HD has been provided in Table 34.1. The prominent oromandibular involvement with

tongue biting is not classical in HD. In this regard, one should consider a couple of conditions, which classically present with movement disorders (chorea and/or dystonia) with prominent oromandibular involvement and tongue/mouth biting and/or injuries, including Lesch–Nyan syndrome and ChAc. The former is, however, less likely in this case given the age at onset (cf. Case 25), while the latter would also fit in with the history of self-injury behaviours, the occurrence of a tonic-clonic seizure and the possible presence of peripheral neuropathy.

Investigations and Diagnosis

Biochemical investigations revealed increased CK (429 IU/L, normal <150) and demonstrated presence of 5 per cent acanthocytes on two occasions. Electrophysiological studies suggested mild myopathy and mild chronic sensory motor axonal neuropathy. A brain MRI revealed a marked volume reduction of the caudate bilaterally with additional frontal atrophy (Figure 35.1). Protein western blot revealed absent chorein, thus confirming the diagnosis of ChAc.

Special Remarks

ChAc is one of the so-called core 'neuroacanthocytosis syndromes with neurodegeneration of the basal ganglia', and is caused by mutations of the VPS13A (vacuolar protein sorting 13 homolog A) gene, encoding for the protein chorein. Indeed, chorein essay has been suggested to be useful for diagnostic procedure in the absence of the genetic analysis. Onset usually occurs in young adulthood, and the clinical features – which include chorea, tics, parkinsonism, eye movement abnormalities, subcortical dementia, and psychiatric features – can mimic HD. Nevertheless, the absence of family history (possibly suggesting a recessive disorder), and the presence of dystonia with prominent orofacial involvement, seizures (present in up to 60 per cent of cases, while only very rarely in HD), self-mutilations, myopathy, and/or neuropathy are useful

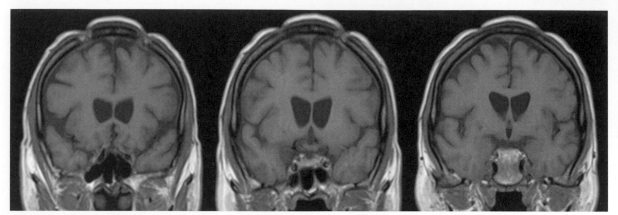

Figure 35.1 Coronal MRI T1-sequences showing caudate nuclei volume loss and mild cortical atrophy.

clues pointing towards the diagnosis of ChAc. Blood tests in patients with chorea–acanthocytosis reveal the presence of acanthocytes in the blood smear and elevated CK. Liver function tests might be abnormal, indicating hepatomegaly. MRI demonstrates progressive caudate atrophy, with a more prominent predilection for the head of the nucleus than that seen in HD. Similar findings can be observed in McLeod syndrome, the other core neuroacanthocytosis syndrome, which is an X-linked disorder due to mutations in the *XK* gene. McLeod is clinically similar to ChAc with involuntary movements that may involve the facio-buccal region but almost never with tongue or lip biting. It can further encompass vocalizations, seizures, peripheral neuropathy, and myopathy. The diagnosis can be confirmed by demonstration of the absence of Kx antigens and a reduction in kell antigens on erythrocytes. Cardiomyopathy and arrhythmia

are distinguishing features and might be a cause of sudden death.

Suggested Readings

Jung HH, Danek A, Walker RH. Neuroacanthocytosis syndromes. *Orphanet J Rare Dis*. 2011:25;6:68.

Martino D, Stamelou M, Bhatia KP. The differential diagnosis of Huntington's disease-like syndromes: 'Red flags' for the clinician. *J Neurol Neurosurg Psychiatry*. 2013;84(6):650–6.

   Video 35.1

There is generalized chorea with truncal movements. He has prominent orobulbar involvement with marked dysarthria with bruxism and tongue biting. His gait is very unstable and lurching.

Case

36

A HD Look-Alike: SCA17

Roberto Erro and Kailash P. Bhatia

Clinical History

This 49-year-old white woman had a 5-year history of walking difficulties, falls, and involuntary movements, which mainly affected her face and limbs. In addition, her family observed speech changes and memory decline whereas she was most troubled by personality changes, with depressive mood and aggressive outbursts. She was carrying a clinical diagnosis of HD, given the strong familial history of a similar disorder occurring in her grandmother, mother, and two of her three siblings.

Examination

On examination, she appeared apathetic, indolent, and cognitively slow. Ocular pursuit was normal, but she had gaze impersistence and difficulty in defixating gaze. Head thrusts were used to initiate saccades. Motor impersistence was seen on tongue protrusion. Speech was jerky. Chorea involving her limbs, face, and trunk was noted, with some additional myoclonic jerks that were not stimulus sensitive (Video 36.1). Repetitive finger and ankle movements were irregular, although the chorea was clearly interfering. Finger–nose testing showed very mild upper limb ataxia. She had a wide-based, stiff gait with occasional freezing. Postural stability was markedly impaired, mainly on backward perturbations. There were no pyramidal or sensory signs.

General Remarks

On the one hand, most clinical features in this patient were compatible with HD, including both the phenotype of chorea, cognitive-behavioural dysfunction, and eye movement abnormalities, and the family history of autosomal dominant inheritance. On the other hand, there were also other clinical findings not entirely consistent with HD including her gait, which had an additional ataxic component. Although walking difficulties

in HD are deemed to represent a 'frontal gait disorder' with a mixture of hypokinetic-rigid and ataxic features, frank ataxia on examination is not classically seen in HD. Most importantly, however, our patient had upper limb ataxia, which again would be against HD. Hence, cerebellar dysfunction in such cases would suggest an alternative diagnosis and the differential diagnosis should be expanded to include the HDL syndromes as well as other HD look-alike conditions (cf. Table 34.1). Among these, the presence of cerebellar dysfunction would pragmatically narrow down the differential diagnosis to two conditions: SCA17 (also referred to as HDL4) and DRPLA. The latter is particularly prevalent in Japan and has been rarely reported in white, African American, and Chinese populations, whereas SCA17 is likely the most common HD-like syndrome in Caucasian populations. Occasionally, other forms of SCA, including SCA1, 2, and 3, may also present with chorea and should be suspected in the presence of cerebellar atrophy on MRI.

Investigations and Diagnosis

A brain MRI revealed cerebellar atrophy, while caudate nuclei size was preserved. Genetic analyses did not reveal mutation in the HD gene as well as in *ATN1*, thus excluding DRPLA. Further genetic testing in the *TBP* gene found a polyglutamine expansion of 46 units and, hence, a diagnosis of SCA17 was made.

Special Remarks

SCA17 accounts for 0.5–1.8 per cent of all HD-like syndromes. Age of onset is usually between 19 and 48 years. Like HD, SCA17 is an autosomal dominant disorder due to a trinucleotide-repeat expansion of the *TBP* gene, which encodes for the TATA-box-binding protein, an important transcription initiation factor. Intergenerational instability, especially during paternal transmission, and anticipation have been reported. Reflecting the broad clinical spectrum, neuropathological findings may vary with a wide participation of the central nervous system involving the cerebellum, cerebral neocortex, basal ganglia (in particular the caudate nucleus), and hippocampus.

Clinically, although cerebellar ataxia is the most frequent clinical feature and found in up to 95 per cent of cases, the phenotype can be markedly heterogeneous. Dystonia and chorea are the two most frequent movement disorders, but parkinsonism can also occur and be associated with abnormal dopaminergic functional imaging. Pyramidal signs occur in more than a third of cases. In addition, dementia, psychiatric disturbances, as well as seizures can occur. In most families, a true HD-like presentation is observed only in a minority of the affected members. However, intra-familial homogeneity has been reported and this was also the case in our patient, who was indeed carrying a clinical diagnosis of HD, also based on the homogenous clinical features of affected family members.

Suggested Readings

Martino D, Stamelou M, Bhatia KP. The differential diagnosis of Huntington's disease-like syndromes: 'red flags' for the clinician. *J Neurol Neurosurg Psychiatry*. 2013;84(6):650–6.

Schneider SA, Walker RH, Bhatia KP. The Huntington's disease-like syndromes: what to consider in patients with a negative Huntington's disease gene test. *Nat Clin Pract Neurol*. 2007;3(9):517–25.

Stevanin G, Brice A. Spinocerebellar ataxia 17 (SCA17) and Huntington's disease-like 4 (HDL4). *Cerebellum*. 2008;7:170–8.

Video 36.1

There is mild chorea in her arms that is also interfering with repetitive finger movements. There is motor impersistence on tongue protrusion. Finger–nose testing shows very mild upper limb ataxia. She has a wide-based gait, and tandem gait is almost impossible.

37

A Newly Recognized HD-Phenocopy Associated with *C9orf72* Expansion

Davina J. Hensman Moss and Sarah J. Tabrizi

Clinical History

This 23-year-old right-handed Caucasian man had a normal birth and early development. Aged 3, he was noted to not interact normally with other children. At the age of 5 years, he was found to have slight difficulties with writing and, aged 6, he was unable to follow basic lessons at primary school. He was hence seen by an educational psychologist, who detected moderate learning difficulties. He therefore subsequently attended a special needs school.

By the age of 8 years, he developed abnormal movements that affected his hands and head, particularly with stress. These involuntary movements worsened over the following years to the point that, at the age of 21 years, they affected his walking, leading to a few falls. Furthermore, he developed aggressive behaviours.

His parents were non-consanguineous and were unaffected. There was, however, a family history of MND on both maternal and paternal sides.

Examination

On examination (Video 37.1), eye movements were found to be abnormal, with poor gaze initiation, impaired pursuit, saccadic hypometria with head thrusts, and reduced vertical up-gaze. There was generalized chorea with oro-buccal involvement and myoclonic movements of the head and neck. There were additional dystonic elements in the limbs, where prominent irregular myoclonic jerks, exacerbated by movement and stimuli, were seen. Gait was slightly broad based, with reduced arm swing and with both arms tending to hold slightly dystonic postures, particularly on the right. He had unsteadiness on tandem walking, but Romberg's test was negative. The remaining neurological examination was normal.

General Remarks

The combination of movement disorders with major chorea and some dystonia, alongside behavioural and cognitive problems, makes the juvenile HD important to exclude (cf. Case 14). However, some features in this case were somewhat unusual for JHD, including the very long duration of cognitive problems and the absence of a dominant family history. Other choreic conditions that can present as early as in the first decade of life include BHC (cf. Case 40) and FDFM (cf. Case 41). They, however, are relatively benign and do not encompass cognitive problems. Despite the age at onset, one should consider the Huntington's disease like syndromes and other genetic conditions that can present with chorea (cf. Table 34.1). Among these, the family history for MND would point towards mutations in the *C9orf72* gene.

Investigations and Diagnosis

Both an extensive set of blood tests and a brain MRI scan were unremarkable. Additional investigations included CSF examination, muscle and skin biopsy, bone marrow aspirate and trephine analysis which were all normal. An EEG revealed a diffuse and nonspecific excess of theta activity. Although the bursts of high-voltage slow activity had a bursting paroxysmal quality, no definite epileptiform activity was seen. On neuropsychological examination, MMSE was 20/28, while the Wechsler Adult Intelligence Scale-Revised was within the defective range consistent with learning difficulties. Genetic testing excluded mitochondrial mutations, DRPLA and HD, and karyotyping was normal, but he was then found to carry an expansion (estimated hexanucleotide repeat size of 3.186) in the *C9orf72* gene.

Special Remarks

Hexanucleotide repeat expansions in the *C9orf72* gene have first been identified in several kindreds with FTD and amyotrophic lateral sclerosis. However, the clinical phenotype associated with *C9orf72* expansions is expanding, and more recently, C9orf72 expansions have been found to be the commonest cause of HD phenocopies. The size of the expansion does not seem to be different from that associated with other clinical presentations due to *C9orf72* expansion, but subjects presenting with chorea and dystonia have a lower age at onset (average of 28 years) compared to those with an FTD phenotype (mean age at onset being 57 years). Besides chorea, *C9orf72* expansion-positive subjects can also show dystonia, myoclonus, and parkinsonism.

The mutation, transmitted in an autosomal dominant fashion, is in a highly conserved gene, with a possible role as a regulator of membrane traffic. The key pathogenic mechanisms are still being determined: both loss and gain of function mechanisms have been proposed. Incomplete penetrance has been previously suggested in *C9orf72*-expanded individuals and, hence, this condition should be suspected also in apparently sporadic cases.

Suggested Readings

Hensman Moss DJ, Poulter M, Beck J, et al. C9orf72 expansions are the most common genetic cause of Huntington disease phenocopies. *Neurology.* 2014;82:292–9.

Rohrer JD, Isaacs AM, Mizielinska S, et al. C9orf72 expansions in frontotemporal dementia and amyotrophic lateral sclerosis. *Lancet Neurol.* 2015;14:291–301.

Wild EJ, Tabrizi SJ. Huntington's disease phenocopy syndromes. *Curr Opin Neurol.* 2007;20:681–7.

Video 37.1

Abnormal eye movements with poor gaze initiation, impaired pursuit, saccadic hypometria with head thrusts, and reduced vertical up-gaze. There is generalized chorea with myoclonic movements of the head and neck. Gait is slightly broad based, with reduced arm swing and with both arms tending to hold slightly dystonic postures. During gait, facial and oro-buccal choreic movements can be seen.

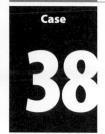

Persistent Chorea Due to Anticholinergics in DYT6

Elena Antelmi, Roberto Erro, and Kailash P. Bhatia

Clinical History

This 68-year-old man, with no family history for any neurological and psychiatric disorders, has been under our care for his dystonic syndrome for a long period. He started suffering from involuntary spasms and abnormal posturing of his neck since his early adolescence. Initially the dystonic spasms involved only his neck. Furthermore, he complained about an irregular head tremor. Progressively the disease worsened and spread to other sites, involving his arm and trunk. He was therefore diagnosed with generalized dystonia. Given the prominent cervical involvement, genetic testing for DYT6 was pursued and he was found to carry an in-frame deletion (c.207_209delCAA) in the *THAP1* gene (cf. Table 16.1).

Over the years, he was treated with botulinum toxin injections for his neck and with trihexyphenidyl (10 mg daily) since his early adulthood, with partial benefit. During the past five years, however, the patient started noting further symptoms, describing recklessness and to be fidgety.

Examination

Besides his dystonia, on examination, there was found to be generalized chorea involving his face, arms (mainly the fingers), legs, and toes. The movements could not be suppressed on volition and were not predictable or patterned and were faster than those usually seen in dystonia (see Video 38.1).

Investigations

Additional investigations in order to exclude both acquired and inherited forms of chorea (copper, ceruplasmin, ferritin, inflammatory markers, autoimmune screening, lactate, pyruvate, acanthocytes, brain MRI, and genetic investigations for DRPLA and HD) were pursued and turned out to be negative.

Remarks

After having excluded a number of inherited and acquired causes of chorea, we interpreted his dyskinesia as a form of tardive chorea and progressively withdrew the trihexyphenidyl. One year after the drug withdrawal, no improvement could be observed as to his choreic movements. Anticholinergic-induced dyskinesia has been rarely reported in dystonic conditions. In these reports, however, drug dosages were higher, and dyskinesia developed within a few days or weeks after the medication had been started and subsided within 2 months after its withdrawal. Nevertheless, the most likely explanation for the dyskinesias occurring in our patient is that they fall under the umbrella of TD, even if this term usually refers to dyskinesia and/or dystonia after neuroleptic exposure (cf. Case 28).

TD have been putatively explained according to different pathophysiological models: dopamine-receptor hypersensitivity, degeneration of striatal interneurons, and maladaptive synaptic plasticity. A possible explanation of the persistence of chorea in our patient may be that while in the previous reports short-term exposure to high-dosage of anti-cholinergic drugs may have induced short-term plastic modulation, in our patient long-term exposure to lower dosage may have prompted long-term maladaptive plasticity. A personal susceptibility due to the *THAP1* mutation cannot be excluded and might have played a role.

Recently, it has been reported that altered dopaminergic responses can unmask an acetylcholine-dependent impairment of corticostriatal synaptic plasticity in animal models of DYT1 dystonia. Given that genes responsible for DYT6 and DYT1 are somewhat related (a role of both genes in dopamine neurotransmission through modulation of D2 dopaminergic receptors has been suggested), an impairment of the cholinergic system may be speculated also in DYT6. This would provide a hypothetical framework to explain why our patient developed persistent chorea even after the drug was discontinued.

Suggested Readings

Maltese M, Martella G, Madeo G, et al. Anticholinergic drugs rescue synaptic plasticity in DYT1 dystonia: Role of M1 muscarinic receptors. *Mov Disord*. 2014;29:1655–65.

Teo JT, Edwards MJ, Bhatia K. Tardive dyskinesia is caused by maladaptive synaptic plasticity: a hypothesis. *Mov Disord*. 2012;27:1205–15.

 Video 38.1

Besides the generalized dystonia, there are generalized choreiform movements involving his face, arms, legs, and toes that are not predictable or patterned.

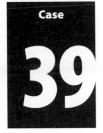

Case

39

Dyskinesia without Levodopa: Long-Term Follow-Up of Mesencephalic Transplant in PD

Roberto Erro, Maria Stamelou, and Kailash P. Bhatia

Clinical History

This 57-year-old man had been diagnosed with PD since the age of 37. Eight years into his disease, he was experiencing increased motor fluctuation, in the forms of wearing-off and sudden-off. He then agreed to receive intrastriatal transplantations of human fetal ventral mesencephalic tissue, as an experimental treatment. Following transplantation, he experienced significant motor benefits, gradually over the first few years. He was able to stop all the dopaminergic treatments including levodopa, within 2 years after the first transplantation, by which time the off periods had virtually ceased. Throughout the post-transplantation course, he never required additional dopaminergic treatments. However, about 3 years after transplantation he started developing dyskinesias, with no reported impact on his daily activities.

Examination

After 12 years after transplant (i.e. 20 years into his disease), he had moderate choreic dyskinesias that affected mainly his lower limbs; he also had abnormal posturing of his neck, trunk, and left foot. He had no bradykinesia on finger tapping, and muscle tone was normal throughout. His gait was mildly unsteady and there were additional dystonic components, but postural reflexes were preserved (see Video 39.1). The remaining neurological examination was unremarkable.

Remarks

Involuntary movements developing after transplantation in PD were first described in the Denver–Columbia clinical trial as mainly dystonic and affecting the arm, head, and neck in up to 15 per cent of transplanted patients. A higher figure was reported in the Tampa–Mount Sinai trial (up to 56 per cent eventually developed dyskinesias), where these hyperkinesias

were described as stereotypic and dystonic and mainly affected the lower parts of the body, hence bearing resemblance with diphasic LID. Reassessment of the 14 patients of the Lund–London trial (which includes the patient presented here) showed choreiform and dystonic dyskinesias, sometimes associated with repetitive and ballistic movements, in up to 43 per cent of the cases. These hyperkinesias, as shown here, appeared as direct consequence of the transplantation of PD within 2 years of the surgery on average, and were not linked to levodopa administration.

Described in general, GID have been reported to be more dystonic, stereotypic, and rhythmic than peak-dose LID and are therefore more comparable to diphasic LID. They were generally mild to moderate but could increase in severity over time. Yet, GID were very different from one patient to another in their manifestation, as well as the time frame over which they developed. It is worth noting that GID has been observed only in patients who show improvements in their PD symptoms, suggesting that such side effects are associated with a functional graft. However, there have also been patients who improved significantly after the transplant but did not develop GID, suggesting that it is not an inevitable consequence of dopamine cell transplantation. Yet, the pathophysiological mechanisms of GID are not clear and further pre-clinical and clinical studies will hopefully clarify which factors are associated with the development of GID, perhaps also shedding light on the pathophysiological underpinnings of LID.

Suggested Readings

Breger LS, Lane EL. L-DOPA and graft-induced dyskinesia: different treatment, same story? *Exp Biol Med (Maywood)*. 2013;238:725–32.

Lane EL, Winkler C. L-DOPA- and graft-induced dyskinesia following transplantation. *Prog Brain Res*. 2012;200:143–68.

Video 39.1

This patient has moderate choreic dyskinesias mainly affecting his lower limbs and additional abnormal posturing of his neck and trunk. His gait is mildly unsteady and there is reduced arm swing. Postural reflexes are preserved.

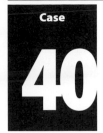

Case

40

Benign Hereditary Chorea due to *TITF-1* Mutations

Roberto Erro and Kailash P. Bhatia

Clinical History

This 35-year-old woman has had long-standing history of a movement disorder since the first year of her life. She was born premature by three weeks and did not feed very well initially. She was noticed to have twitching movements of her limbs right from her birth. This was initially thought to be possibly related to birth anoxia. Moreover, initial motor milestones were delayed and she tended to fall. However, over a period of time both her movement disorder and her walking difficulty seemed to improve and, in fact, she did not report at the consultation major issues with regard to either of the involuntary movements or of gait. The main reason to seek medical advices was in relation to the fact that her daughter, now aged 6, showed similar disturbances since her birth, even though somewhat more pronounced than in the mother.

Examination

On examination (see Video 40.1), ocular movements and cranial nerve were found to be normal. There was mild motor impersistence of the tongue when protruded outside the mouth. Moreover, she had bilateral chorea with superimposed dystonic posturing of her limbs. Her gait was minimally affected by a mixture of chorea and dystonia. There were no pyramidal or cerebellar features, and the rest of the neurological examination was normal. The clinical phenotype in her daughter was similar in that she also had a mixture of chorea and dystonia, but with more marked dystonic gait and a tendency to fall.

General Remarks

Pragmatically, there are only two conditions that should be considered when facing with a patient with such a long-standing, benign (i.e. apparently non-progressive), condition featuring mainly distal chorea or chorea-like movements: BHC and myoclonus-dystonia. These two disorders can be sometimes

difficult to distinguish and such a difficulty reflects the clinical challenge in discriminating between minimal distal chorea and myoclonus. Both conditions have an autosomal dominant inheritance, early age at onset and minimal progression (cf. Case 52). In our patients, the clinical improvement over time, the absence of psychiatric features (cf. Case 52) as well as the specific phenotype, which was clinically deemed to encompass chorea rather than myoclonus, favoured the diagnosis of BHC.

Investigations and Diagnosis

Standard blood investigations, including thyroid function, were unremarkable. Brain MRI was normal in both patients. Genetic screening for *TITF-1* mutations revealed the presence of a previously unpublished heterozygous A>G substitution at nucleotide 701 and predicted to change a Glutamine with an Arginine at position 202. The mutated Glutamine is an evolutionary highly conserved amino acid in the TTF1 homeodomain, and such a variation was predicted to be likely pathogenic. The diagnosis of BHC due to a *TITF-1* mutation was hence confirmed.

Special Remarks

BHC is a rare (prevalence of around 2 in 10 millions) autosomal dominant movement disorder characterized by a non-progressive form of chorea and absence of other major neurological symptoms. The condition is due to mutations in the *TITF-1* gene on chromosome 14q (encoding the thyroid transcription factor-1), and its penetrance is estimated to be complete in men and 75 per cent in women. This gene is involved in the function of thyroid and lung and, in fact, affected individuals may also have pulmonary disease and/or congenital hypothyroidism. For this reason, BHC is described as part of the 'brain–lung–thyroid syndrome'. Age at onset is usually before 5 years and often within the first 2 years of life, but despite this can vary and cases with onset in late childhood and adolescence have been described. Delayed motor milestones – specifically late walking, clumsiness, and frequent falls – characterize affected children, but these features tend to improve over time. Speech and intellect are normally unaffected or minimally affected. Progression during adulthood is extremely rare and life expectancy is normal. However, the condition can show remarkable intra- and inter-familial phenotypic heterogeneity. Atypical features that have been occasionally reported include dysarthria and 'major' gait disturbances, mental impairment, or axial dystonia.

A general therapeutic treatment is not available. Levodopa has been reported to be effective with regard to gait difficulties, whereas tetrabenazine may be an option to treat disabling chorea. As stated earlier, however, the condition is benign by definition and tends to improve over time in many patients.

A final consideration concerns the genetic heterogeneity of BHC. Indeed, not all cases clinically diagnosed with BHC are tested positive for *TITF-1* mutations, suggesting that other genes can produce a similar phenotype (cf. Case 41).

Suggested Readings

Gras D, Jonard L, Roze E, et al. Benign hereditary chorea: phenotype, prognosis, therapeutic outcome and long term follow-up in a large series with new mutations in the TITF1/NKX2-1 gene. *J Neurol Neurosurg Psychiatry*. 2012;83:956–62.

Veneziano L, Parkinson MH, Mantuano E, Frontali M, Bhatia KP, Giunti P. A novel de novo mutation of the TITF1/NKX2-1 gene causing ataxia, benign hereditary chorea, hypothyroidism and a pituitary mass in a UK family and review of the literature. *Cerebellum*. 2014;13:588–95.

 Video 40.1

There is motor impersistence on tongue protrusion. Generalized choreic movements are seen mainly in the upper limbs but also in the lower ones and toes. There is also mild dystonic posturing of the fingers bilaterally.

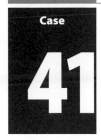

Case

41

Another Cause of Benign Hereditary Chorea due to *ADCY5* Mutations

Roberto Erro and Kailash P. Bhatia

Clinical History

This 36-year-old man had onset in the first year of life. After an uncomplicated birth, he progressively developed brief choreic movements that affected the face and the four limbs. These movements were present at rest, but could be exacerbated by excitement, stress, and tiredness. There were no other complaints, and his milestones were otherwise normal. Nevertheless, his symptoms slowly progressed and around the age of 18, he further developed painful spasms of the four limbs, characteristically present upon awakening. He also complained about abnormal posturing of his neck and arms. Furthermore, his speech articulation started being affected and impairing his social relationships.

Of note, his father, aged 64, had similar involuntary movements starting age 1, but they were far less prominent and did not encompass abnormal posturing. He in fact never sought medical advice for himself. When they were first examined, a working diagnosis of BHC was made.

Examination

Clinical examination (see Video 41.1) revealed dysarthric speech and severe abnormal involuntary movements comprising generalized chorea with facial grimacing and dystonic elements. Both chorea and dystonia were present at rest, but were more evident on posture and action. Eye movements were abnormal with gaze impersistence and use of head thrust to initiate saccades. Gait was unsteady with both choreic and dystonic features, but cerebellar testing was normal.

The involuntary movements in the father consisted of minimal generalized chorea, with no dystonic features. Besides chorea, he had tandem walking difficulties, but cerebellar testing was otherwise normal. The remaining examination was normal.

General Remarks

BHC is a rare clinical syndrome characterized by early onset (infancy or early childhood) chorea with little clinical progression and absence of other major neurological deficits, including cognitive decline. In 2002, heterozygous mutations in the *TITF-1* gene (also known as *NKX2-1*) have been associated with the autosomal dominant form of BHC (cf. Case 40). Since then, a number of pedigree have been described with mutations in this gene and it is now well recognized that *TTF-1* mutations lead to a complex multisystem disease (also termed brain–lung–thyroid syndrome) that, besides chorea, can additionally encompass hypotonia, neurodevelopmental delay, learning disabilities, dystonia, myoclonus, tics, and ataxia. Moreover, being TTF-1 (i.e. thyroid transcriptor factor 1) crucial for both thyroid and lung development, hypothyroidism, and pulmonary defects can be observed in affected individuals (cf. Case 40). However, a number of patients clinically diagnosed with BHC do not carry *TTF-1* mutations, suggesting genetic heterogeneity of this clinical syndrome.

Investigations and Diagnosis

Basic diagnostic investigations – including brain MRI, CSF analysis, acanthocytes, antistreptolysin titer, copper, ceruloplasmin, and α-fetoprotein – were unremarkable. Both the index case and his father were found negative for mutations in the *TTF-1* gene and for the HD triplet expansion. Whole-exome sequencing revealed the c.1252C>T mutation in the *ADCY5* gene, which has been associated with a spectrum of clinical manifestations including a syndrome referred to as Familial Dyskinesia and Facial Myokymia (FDFM). Although our patients never displayed facial dyskinesias, an EMG of periorbital and perioral regions was performed, but failed to show either myokymia or other signs of motor neuron hyperexcitability.

Special Remarks

Prior to the identification of facial myokymia as one of the core features of this disorder, the original FDFM kindred had been initially diagnosed with BHC. As at present, few families and sporadic cases have been reported with mutations in this gene, allowing a better definition of the phenotype. Onset is early in life between the first year of life and early adolescence, and the disorder is mainly characterized by chorea, but axial hypothonia, dystonia, pyramidal signs, and also delayed milestones have been reported. In some cases, dystonia can be prominent and overshadow choreic features. Paroxysmal attacks of chorea and/or ballism have been described. A distinctive feature of this disorder is the possible presence of prominent periorbital and perioral facial dyskinesias that were initially erroneously thought to represent myokymias.

Although *ADCY5*-related phenotype bears resemblance to BHC associated with *TTF-1* mutations, there are a number of features that can aid the differential diagnosis. First, the extra-neurological involvement can encompass thyroid and pulmonary dysfunction in individuals with *TTF-1* mutations. ADCY5 is instead highly expressed in the cardiac tissue, and in fact cardiac involvement has been described in some patients with this condition. Second, the clinical progression between the two disorders seems to be different, with *TTF-1* mutation carriers remaining stable and minimally affected over time, whereas patients with *ADCY5* mutations seem to progress and develop other features such as prominent dystonia. Third, other neurological abnormalities, including mild ocular and gait abnormalities, are often present in this condition, while they are seldom seen in *TTF-1*-related BHC.

Although this disorder has been first termed as FDFM, a suspicion of *ADCY5*-related disorder should be raised when facing patients with a relatively pure BHC-like presentation, regardless of the presence of facial dyskinesias. Worth of note, the phenotypic spectrum of *ADCY5*-related disorder is constantly increasing with some patients presenting with isolated dystonia, paroxysmal dyskinesias, and more complex syndrome with axial hypotonia and myoclonus.

Suggested Readings

Carapito R, Paul N, Untrau M, et al. A De Novo ADCY5 mutation causes early-onset autosomal dominant chorea and dystonia. *Mov Disord*. 2015;30:423–7.

Chen DH, Méneret A, Friedman JR., et al. ADCY5-related dyskinesia: broader spectrum and genotype-phenotype correlations. *Neurology*. 2015;85:2026–3.

Mencacci NE, Erro R, Wiethoff S. et al. ADCY5 mutations are another cause of benign hereditary chorea. *Neurology*. 2015;85:80–8.

Video 41.1

There is generalized chorea with superimposed dystonic posturing, with clear torticollis to the left. Gait is unsteady with both choreiform and dystonic features.

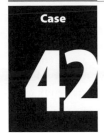

Essential Tremor

Roberto Erro and Kailash P. Bhatia

Clinical History

This now 72-year-old right-handed man had a normal birth and milestones and has been generally in good health. He sought medical advice for shaking of both hands mainly on action or when holding objects. He mentioned that his tremor probably started about 8 years earlier, but it was only in the last year that he felt that it was interfering with some of his activities of daily life such as writing. The tremor was more on the right side. There was no clear family history and he did not find that his tremor improved with ingestion of alcohol.

Examination

On examination (Video 42.1), eye movements and cranial nerves were found to be normal. There was no tremor at rest, while he had a moderate bilateral postural tremor, which was slightly more pronounced on the right than the left. There was also a moderate bilateral action tremor that increased in amplitude when coming closer to a target. He also had a writing tremor. There was no dystonia, and repetitive finger and foot movements were deemed normal, despite the fact that it was difficult to judge whether there was indeed some slowness since tremor took over the frequency of the tapping. His tremor was neither distractible nor entrainable. While walking was normal and arm swing preserved, tandem walking was mildly unsteady, but possible. There were no other neurological abnormalities.

General Remarks

There are several conditions that should be considered in the differential diagnosis of tremor (Table 42.1), but a careful history taking (patients should be screened for medications, drugs of abuse, and alcohol consumption) can exclude some of these conditions on clinical grounds.

When facing with a tremulous patient, a typical approach would be to distinguish tremor by when it appears (e.g. rest, postural, action), distribution, and frequency. In our patient, tremor was postural/kinetic with an additional intention component and involved the upper limbs, with a slight asymmetry. Such features (i.e. absence of a rest component along with the lack of bradykinesia) would make PD less likely. Similarly, the absence of overt dystonia would rule out a dystonic tremor. The bilateral distribution would instead render a structural lesion unlikely, while the absence of other neurological symptoms as well as the benign course would exclude other neurodegenerative conditions that can present with tremor.

Investigations and Diagnosis

Standard blood investigations, including thyroid and liver function, were normal. A brain MRI disclosed mild general atrophy in keeping with age. Electrophysiological testing showed that tremor frequency was at about 6.5 Hz in both postural and action conditions, with an alternating activity in antagonist muscles. Loading test with 1 kg mass very modestly reduced tremor amplitude, and had no effect on its frequency, excluding an enhanced physiological tremor and thus leading to a diagnosis of ET.

Special Remarks

ET is mostly an autosomal dominant condition, the incidence of which peaks in a bimodal fashion with age of onset common during adolescence/early adulthood or when older than 60 years. Recently, the entity of 'aging-related tremor' has been proposed to account for the second peak of ET. Aging-related tremor (which should be considered in our case given his age at onset), starts by definition later in life and is accompanied by subtle signs of aging both cognitively and physically. It might hence represent a different disease entity altogether within the ET syndromes.

Studies of twins have reported higher, but not absolute, concordance rates in monozygotic twins. Yet, no

Table 42.1 Commonest Causes of Arm Tremor

Type of Tremor	Conditions
Rest tremor	PD
	Drug-induced parkinsonism
	Atypical parkinsonism (rare)
	Adult onset dystonia
	SCAs (especially SCA2 and SCA3)
	Psychogenic tremor
	ET (extremely rare)
Postural tremor	Enhanced physiological tremor
	Drugs/toxins
	Systemic diseases (liver dysfunction, hyperthyroidism, Cushing's syndrome)
	ET
	Neuropathy
	Dystonia
	Task-specific tremor
	PD (usually re-emergent)
	MSA (up to 60% of patients)
	SCAs (especially SCA12)
	Fragile X
	OT
	Psychogenic tremor
Kinetic tremor	Cerebellar disease*
	Holmes tremor*
	WD*
	ET (uncommon)
	Psychogenic

* Rest and postural tremor may occur.

definitive association with any genes has been found to date, although certain variants in the *LINGO1* and *FUS* genes have been found to confer a higher risk for ET. The failure in finding causative genes for ET probably relies on the fact that there are no reliable biomarkers for tremor and, as such, it has been probably over-diagnosed.

ET is primarily a monosymptomatic condition affecting the hands. The Movement Disorder Society Consensus Statement on Tremor in fact defines ET as a bilateral, largely symmetrical, postural, or kinetic tremor affecting hands and forearms, with or without an additional head involvement in the absence of abnormal posturing. On the contrary, exclusion criteria include other neurological signs, especially dystonia, and the presence of isolated position-specific or task-specific tremor. Nevertheless, it has been demonstrated that ET patients can have subtle cerebellar signs on examination, including tandem gait difficulties (as our patient had), with normal walking unaffected. This evidence is in line with the hypothesis that ET arises from the disruption of the olivo-cerebello-rubral pathway. Improvement with ethanol and primidone (as outlined earlier) implicate a possible role of GABAergic transmission (i.e. activation GABA receptors and release of GABA by endogenous or pharmacological modulators).

ET often worsens slowly over many years, but usually does not cause marked functional impairment. It often improves after alcohol, and may be helped by β-blockers, primidone, gabapentin, and topiramate in some cases.

Suggested Readings

Deuschl G, Bain P, Brin M. Consensus statement of the Movement Disorder Society on Tremor. Ad Hoc Scientific Committee. *Mov Disord*. 1998;13 Suppl 3:2–23.

Quinn NP, Schneider SA, Schwingenschuh P, Bhatia KP. Tremor-some controversial aspects. *Mov Disord*. 2011;26:18–23.

Schrag A, Münchau A, Bhatia KP, Quinn NP, Marsden CD. Essential tremor: an overdiagnosed condition? *J Neurol*. 2000;247:955–9.

Video 42.1

There is no tremor at rest. A fine symmetrical tremor of his arms can be seen on posture, with no evidence of dystonia. The tremor is more evident on action (finger–nose test, writing, pouring water from one glass to another).

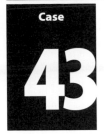

Case

43

Rest Tremor and Scans without Evidence of Dopaminergic Deficit (SWEDD)

Roberto Erro and Kailash P. Bhatia

Clinical History

This 75-year-old right-handed woman with no family history for any neurological disorders and who had been generally in good health for all her life, came to see us for the development of a right-sided arm tremor, which started about one year earlier. She previously consulted a general neurologist who, suspecting the development of PD, requested a DaT-Scan, which turned out to be entirely normal. There were no other major complaints apart from her tremor, which was present at rest as well as when holding objects or on action. Her writing had become in fact difficult and she mentioned that feeding and other activities of daily life were affected as well. On specific questioning, she mentioned that she had mildly slowed down, but she attributed this to her age.

Examination

On examination (Video 43.1), she was found to be hypomimic with reduced blink rate. She had a resting tremor of her right hand and a bilateral (but asymmetric) postural tremor with no re-emergence. On posture, the tremor increased in amplitude when she was asked to flex her elbows. In such a position, a mild abnormal posturing of her left arm was evident. She also had bilateral action tremor on the finger–nose test. Furthermore, she had a very mild abnormal posture of her head, the latter being slightly tilted to the right and turned to the left. The remaining neurological examination, including gait and finger/foot tapping, was entirely normal.

General Remarks and Diagnosis

Although a suspicion of PD in this case is reasonable given the combination of asymmetric rest tremor and hypomimia, there are also other clinical features, which are instead suggestive of another condition masquerading as PD. Indeed, the crucial hallmark of the latter is bradykinesia (cf. Case 1) that was not present

in this case. Moreover, this patient had no re-emergent tremor (which is deemed to be classic of PD) and her gait (and arm swing) was normal. Finally, she had abnormal posturing of her head and arm and it is now increasingly recognized that patients with adult-onset dystonia can manifest with a phenotype resembling that of PD. In this regard, a previous DaT-Scan was found to be normal, thus definitively excluding PD according to current criteria for PD. On the contrary, it has to be remarked that sometimes the clinical diagnosis of dystonia can be challenging and that there are no definite biomarkers for dystonia. In this case, however, abnormal posturing was quite clear, especially in her arms and, therefore, she was eventually diagnosed with adult-onset tremulous dystonia.

Special Remarks

A number of patients (up to 14 per cent), enrolled in drug trials of neuroprotection for PD and subjected to DaT-Scan, were subsequently found to have normal scans. Their scans were hence labelled 'scans without evidence for dopaminergic deficit' (SWEDD), and this term has been widely used since, also in clinical practice. Although some authors suggested that patients with SWEDD could represent a (benign) subtype of PD, there has been increasing evidence that a number of different conditions can mimic PD. Specifically, it has been shown that patients with adult-onset dystonia can have, in addition to an asymmetric or unilateral rest tremor of the hands, hypomimia, reduced arm swing, and/or jaw tremor and even an impairment of finger tapping similar to PD patients (but without true decrement), thus rendering the differential diagnosis with PD challenging in individual cases.

Described in general, however, there are some clinical clues related to the tremor itself, including position/task specificity, jerkiness, absence of re-emergent tremor, presence of tremor-flurries and thumb hyperextension, which would be fairly typical for dystonic tremor and are instead not classically seen in PD. The diagnosis of dystonic tremor, however, relies on the presence of overt dystonia on examination (as in this case) and clinicians should hence carefully look for dystonic features, also in non-tremulous body segments. However, it must be remembered there are a number of different causes accounting for subjects with SWEDD such as HD, FXTAS, and psychogenic parkinsonism.

Suggested Readings

Erro R, Rubio-Agusti I, Saifee TA, et al. Rest and other types of tremor in adult-onset primary dystonia. *J Neurol Neurosurg Psychiatry*. 2014;85:965–8.

Erro R, Schneider SA, Stamelou M, Quinn NP, Bhatia KP. What do patients with scans without evidence of dopaminergic deficit (SWEDD) have? New evidence and continuing controversies. *J Neurol Neurosurg Psychiatry*. 2016;87:319–23.

Schneider SA, Edwards MJ, Mir P, et al. Patients with adult-onset dystonic tremor resembling parkinsonian tremor have scans without evidence of dopaminergic deficit (SWEDDs). *Mov Disord*. 2007;22:2210–5.

 Video 43.1

She is hypomimic. There is a rest tremor of her right hand. A bilateral postural tremor of her arms is shown, with no re-emergence. There is no bradykinesia.

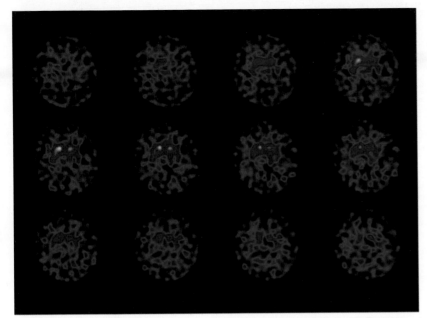

Figure 2.1 DaT-Scan SPECT showing reduced uptake in the posterior putamen (left>right) and relative sparing of the caudate nuclei.

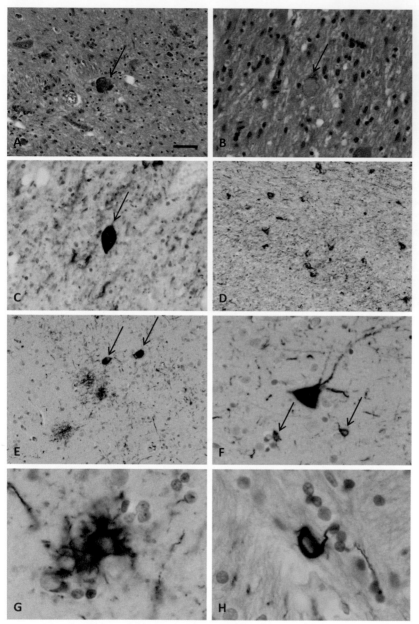

Figure 5.1 Histological examination showed neuropathological changes of progressive supranuclear palsy. In the substantia nigra there was moderate loss of dopaminergic pigmented neurons, and some residual neurons contained basophilic neurofibrillary tangles (A, arrow indicates a neuron with a neurofibrillary tangle). In the subthalamic nucleus there was gliosis and neuronal loss with neurofibrillary tangles in several surviving neurons (B, arrow indicates a neuron containing a neurofibrillary tangle), confirmed by positive staining using tau immunohistochemistry (C, arrow). In the cerebellar white matter there were numerous coiled bodies and threads (D). Tau positive structures in the frontal cortex (E and F) included neurofibrillary tangles (E, arrows) and tufted astrocytes (E) while higher magnification revealed several coiled bodies (F, arrows). In the caudate nucleus typical tufted astrocytes were found (G) and there were numerous coiled bodies in the internal capsule (H).

(Bar in A represents 50 μm in A, D, & E; 25 μm in B, C, & F; 10 μm in G & H. Haematoxylin and eosin: A & B. Tau immunohistochemistry: C-H.)

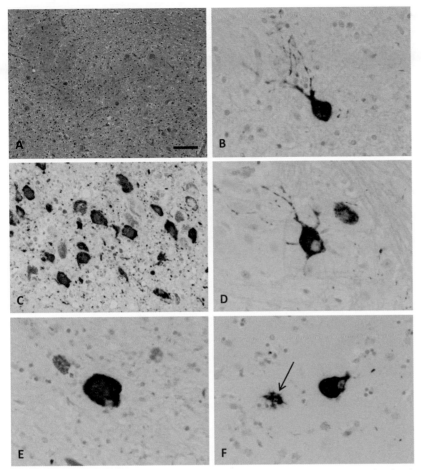

Figure 6.1 Histological examination confirmed neuronal and glial tau pathology with a distribution and type typical of progressive supranuclear palsy. In the dentate nucleus there was gliosis and mild loss of neurons (A), a number of the remaining neurons contained tau immunoreactive neurofibrillary tangles (B). The locus coeruleus was well preserved but contained numerous neurofibrillary tangles (C) and these were also present in modest numbers in the pontine nuclei (D). The substantia nigra showed severe loss of pigmented neurons with neurofibrillary tangles in several remaining neurons (E). There were scattered neurofibrillary tangles and tufted astrocytes (arrow) in the caudate nucleus (F).

(Bar in A represents 100 μm in A; 50 μm in C; 25 μm in B, D, E, & F. Haematoxylin and eosin: A. Tau immunohistochemistry: B – F.)

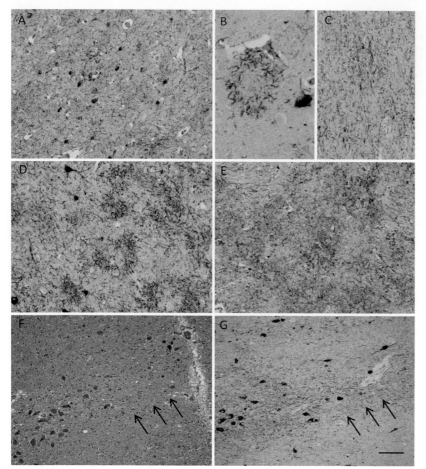

Figure 7.2 Tau immunohistochemistry demonstrates numerous pretangles, neurofibrillary tangles, and neuropil threads in the prefrontal cortex (A). Astrocytic plaques, which are one of the diagnostic criteria of corticobasal degeneration, were readily found in cerebral cortices and subcortical nuclei in this case (B). Tau-positive neurites and threads were numerous in the subcortical white matter (C). The tau pathology with numerous neuropil threads and astrocytic plaques was severe in both the amygdala (D) and caudate nucleus (E). The loss of neuromelaning-containing neurons (arrows) was of moderate degree in the pars compacta of the substantia nigra (F), but most of the remaining neurons contained either pretangles or neurofibrillary tangles (G).

(Bar on G represents 160 microns on F and G, 80 microns on A, C-E, and 40 microns on B. A-E and G: tau immunohistochemistry (AT8 antibody); F: haematoxylin and eosin stain.)

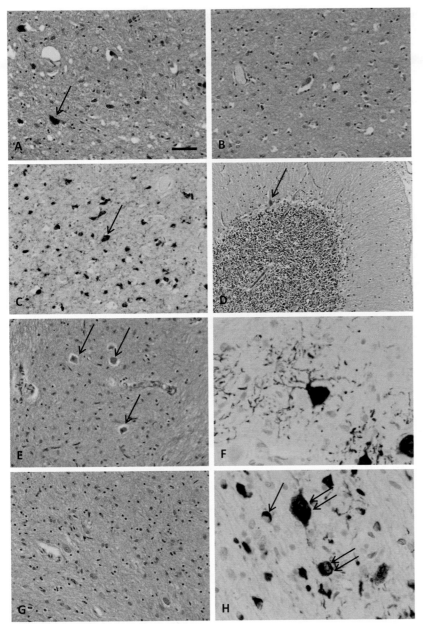

Figure 8.2 Histological examination showed typical features of multiple system atrophy with involvement of striatonigral and olivopontocerebellar regions. There was marked loss of pigmented neurons in the substantia nigra with scattered clusters of neuromelanin in the neuropil (A, arrow indicates a residual pigmented neuron). In the putamen there was moderate neuronal loss (B) and α-synuclein immunohistochemistry demonstrated frequent neuronal cytoplasmic inclusions (arrow) and glial cytoplasmic inclusions (C). Only sparse residual Purkinje cells were present in the cerebellum (D, arrow). The inferior olivary nucleus was gliotic with moderate neuronal loss (E, arrows indicate residual neurons) and many residual neurons contained neuronal cytoplasmic inclusions (F). There was also moderate loss of neurons in the pontine nuclei (G) where there were frequent glial cytoplasmic inclusions (arrow), and neurons often contained both cytoplasmic and nuclear inclusions (double arrow) (H).

(Bar in A represents 100 μm in D; 50 μm in A, B, C, E, & G; 25 μm in F & H. Haematoxylin and eosin: A, B, D, E & G. α-Synuclein immunohistochemistry: C, F, & H.)

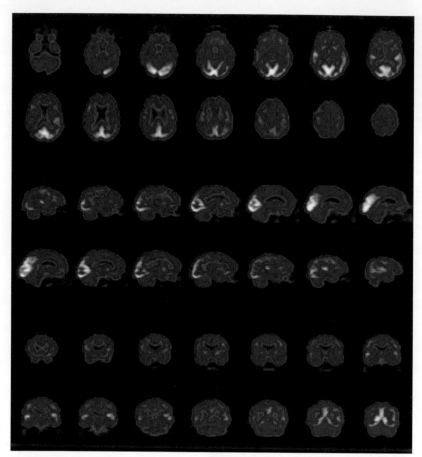

Figure 15.2 FDG-PET scan of the brain demonstrating reduced tracer uptake in the frontal and right parietal lobe.

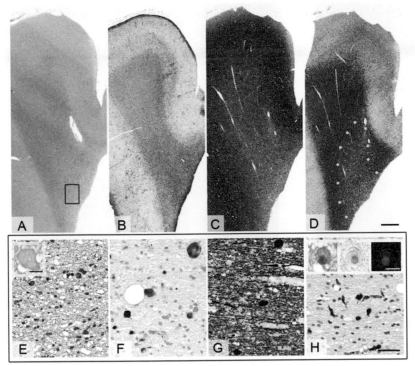

Figure 15.3 Full thickness brain biopsy. The Hematoxylin and Eosin (H&E) stain (A), immunostaining for glial fibrillary acid protein (B), axons (neurofilament cocktail), (C) and myelin (Luxol fast blue/cresyl violet) (D) shows a mild pallor of the myelin and reduction of axon density towards the deep white matter (separated by a yellow dotted line in D) where frequent axonal spheroids are seen (inset in E). The axonal spheroids label with antibodies for neurofilaments (E), amyloid precursor protein (F), and ubiquitin (G). Increased numbers of CD68 positive microglial cells are present in the deeper white matter (H), which show yellow–light brown cytoplasm on H&E and negative control sections and appear blue when viewed as a negative colour inversion image (insets in H). *(Scale bar: 1mm in A-D, 5μm in E-H, 10μm insets in E and H.)*

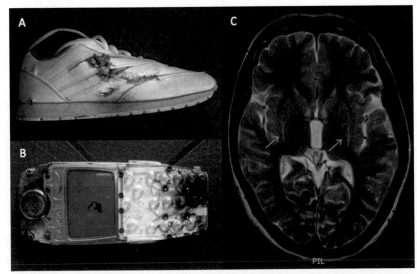

Figure 29.1 (A) Left shoe with a hole, through which the lightning exited; (B) Burnt-out mobile phone that our patient was holding when struck by the lightning; (C) Axial T2-sequence showing bilateral hyperintensity (mineralization) in the posterior putamen (arrows).

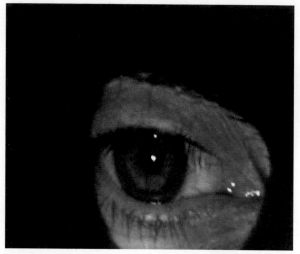

Figure 45.1 Kayser–Fleischer ring with copper deposition in Descemet's membrane, leading to brown discolouration at the outer margin of the cornea.

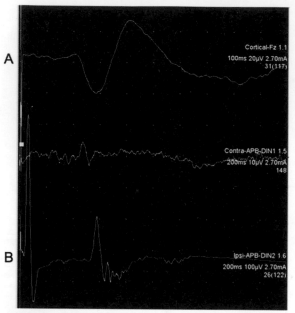

Figure 58.1 (A) Giant SSEPs over the left hemisphere; (B) presence of the C-reflex, elicited after the stimulation of the median nerve.

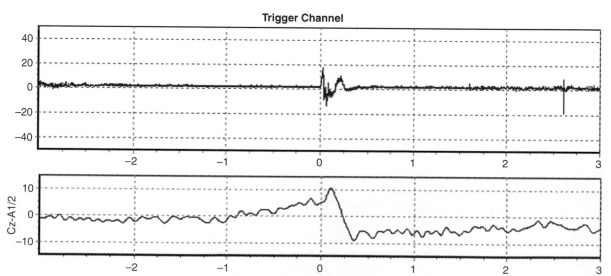

Figure 60.1 Jerk-locked EEG back averaging showing a negative shift with amplitude of more than 5 microvolts over the central cortical areas, starting about 1 second before the jerks (i.e. the bereitschaftspotential).

Neuropathic Tremor

Roberto Erro and Kailash P. Bhatia

Clinical History

A 52-year-old right-handed man with no family history came to see us for shaking of both his hands, which had started about 2 years earlier. His tremor was initially present intermittently and mainly when holding objects, but had progressively worsened over time. Tremor did not improve with alcohol. He further mentioned that over the past 3 or 4 years he was feeling pins and needles distally in his lower limbs. His past medical history was of no relevance.

Examination

On examination (Video 44.1), a fairly symmetrical tremor of his hands when keeping his arms outstretched and on action (i.e. writing a sentence and drawing a spiral) was noticed. The tremor was neither distractible nor entrainable. There was neither tremor at rest nor bradykinesia or abnormal posturing. His feet dorsiflexion was found to be weak and deep tendon reflexes were barely elicitable in his lower limbs. Furthermore, he has reduced pin-pick sensation up to ankles bilaterally. Nevertheless, walking was judged to be normal. The remaining neurological examination was unremarkable.

General Remarks

A list of the most common conditions accounting for tremor has been provided in Table 42.1. In our patient, there were on examination some features that have narrowed the differential diagnosis. In fact, the presence of motor and sensory dysfunction in the lower limbs and absent tendon reflexes were indicative of a peripheral neuropathy and it is known that tremor, especially on posture, can be present in a number of different types of inflammatory neuropathies.

Investigations and Diagnosis

Standard blood investigations, including thyroid and liver function, and a brain MRI were normal. A nerve conduction study revealed reduced conduction velocities, prolonged distal motor and F-wave latencies, and presence of conduction blocks in more than three nerves, thus leading to the diagnosis of CIDP. As stated elsewhere, there are no biomarkers for the differential diagnosis of tremulous disorders, but we would not invoke another different condition (such as ET) to explain the tremor in our patient and rather believed this was part and parcel of his CIDP.

Special Remarks

It has been reported that the majority of patients with inflammatory neuropathies have tremor. One study has shown that up to 65 per cent of these patients, taken as a whole, have tremor, but this estimate rises to up to 80 per cent if one considers only patients with IgM paraproteinaemic neuropathy. However, tremor can be present in any other inflammatory neuropathies, including CIDP, multifocal motor neuropathy with conduction block, and in the recovery phase of Guillain–Barré syndrome. There are no prospective studies showing tremor onset in relation to neuropathy onset, but it is generally assumed that the latter always manifests first. Our patient indeed complained about pins and needles in his lower extremities that started at least a couple of year before his tremor. Yet, he only sought medical advices for the latter, suggesting that tremor can be the most disturbing feature of neuropathy in some patients.

The pathophysiology of tremor occurring in the context of neuropathy is not entirely clear. In fact, no relationship seems to exist between the development and intensity of tremor and the severity of the neuropathy, proprioceptive loss, weakness, or fatigue. Moreover, it has to be determined why only a subset, yet the majority, of such patients develop tremor. The evidence that loading test does not affect tremor frequency in these patients promotes the hypothesis of an important central mechanism (perhaps driven by the cerebellum) in generating the tremor.

Tremor in inflammatory neuropathies can be as disabling as the underlying neuropathy itself. Unfortunately, it is usually refractory to any treatments commonly used for tremor, and only in a small number of cases it improves with treatment of the underlying neuropathy. A few cases have been reported on, who improved after thalamic DBS.

Suggested Readings

Saifee TA, Schwingenschuh P, Reilly MM, et al. Tremor in inflammatory neuropathies. *J Neurol Neurosurg Psychiatry*. 2013;84:1282–7.

Smith IS. Tremor in peripheral neuropathy. In: Findley LJ, Koller WC, eds. *Handbook of tremor disorders*. New York: Marcel Dekker, Inc, 1995:12.

Video 44.1

There is a bilateral, symmetric postural fine tremor of the upper limbs with no dystonic posturing, while no tremor is seen at rest and on action.

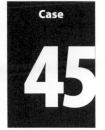

Wilson's Disease Misdiagnosed as ET

Roberto Erro and Kailash P. Bhatia

Clinical History

This 38-year-old man with no family history had a normal birth, early milestones, and normal scholastic achievements. He has been in the army since the age of 28 and served in Iraq and Cyprus. Aged 35, he had his first symptoms, namely that of tremor, which he noticed when he was feeding his son. This was initially very minimal and not interfering with his day-to-day activities. In fact, after a diagnosis of ET was made, no treatment was suggested. However, aged 37 he had a bad flu lasting for about 3 weeks and, according to him, his symptoms markedly worsened since. His writing became affected and he had difficulty carrying cups of tea. Moreover, his tremor spread to his head. At this stage, he was put on propranolol (80 mg daily), without any noticeable differences and was therefore sent to us for a second opinion.

On further questioning, he denied any benefit from alcohol and also any family history for tremor. There has been no further progression of his symptoms. However, his mother mentioned that since he had come back from Iran (5 years earlier) his eye blue colour was turning brown, as if some 'desert dust had gone into his eyes'.

Examination

On examination (Video 45.1), extra ocular movements were found to be full and normal. There was a head tremor. He had a mild resting tremor of his arms and a bilateral postural tremor of his arms when keeping them outstretched, with some mold posturing of his fingers. There was dysmetria and terminal tremor on the index–nose test, more on the right than the left. Furthermore, he has difficulty on alternating cerebellar tasks. There were no other neurological abnormalities.

General Remarks

Although his former diagnosis of ET would have been reasonable (despite a number of features arguing against ET such as the age at onset, absence of family history, and no response to alcohol; cf. Case 42), there were on examination, and also by history, a few clues suggesting an alternative condition. First, ET tremor does not feature a resting component or any dystonic elements. Second, head tremor is hardly seen in ET, at least early during the disease course. Third, although ET is somehow supposed to reflect a cerebellar dysfunction (cf. Case 42), gross cerebellar abnormalities on examination do not fit with ET and should prompt to look for another condition. Finally, there was the report of his eye changing colour, which was indeed very useful in guiding the subsequent investigations.

Investigations and Diagnosis

Free serum copper was 2 µg/dL and ceruloplasmin was 0.05 g/L, both abnormally low. A ocular examination showed Kayser–Fleischer rings bilaterally (Figure 45.1). A brain MRI was performed which showed bilateral T2 hyperintensity involving the putamen and the thalamus, bilaterally. Moreover, the characteristic 'giant panda sign' was noted in the brainstem (cf. Case 11 and Figure 11.1A). A genetic test was pursued and he was confirmed compound heterozygous for the c.C3008T mutation in exon 13 and the c.C3207A mutation in exon 14 of the *ATP7B* gene, thus confirming a diagnosis of WD.

Special Remarks

While WD has been described more in general in Case 11, we would here focus on its tremulous form. Historically, neurologic WD presentations have been divided into four primary subgroups, including parkinsonian, tremor and dysarthria predominant ('pseudosclerotic'), dystonic, and choreic. The actual frequency of such phenotypes varies significantly in different studies, but it seems that the pseudosclerotic variant is one of the commonest along with the dystonic variant. Tremor has been in fact reported to be present in up to 55 per cent of cases. Although widely known, the wing-beating

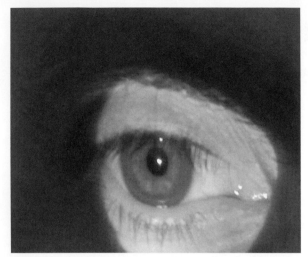

Figure 45.1 Kayser–Fleischer ring with copper deposition in Descemet's membrane, leading to brown discolouration at the outer margin of the cornea. A black and white version of this figure will appear in some formats. For the colour version, please refer to the plate section.

tremor of WD does not appear to be the most frequent tremor type. However, when present, classic wing-beating tremor and/or flapping tremor in combination with dysarthria strongly suggests the diagnosis of WD. The classic posture-induced wing-beating tremor is thought to be associated with lesions of the dentadorubrothalamic pathway, and features a low frequency, high amplitude, proximal upper extremity tremor elicited by holding the arms extended laterally or with the arms held in front with flexed elbows and palms facing downwards. The wing-beating tremor is typified by increasing amplitude with increased duration of posture holding.

However, other types of tremor, including rest, action, or intention tremor, can occur. The kinetic tremor is most frequently a distal upper extremity tremor, with low amplitude and medium-to-high frequency, thus generating the potential for ET misdiagnosis, as in our case. This might be one of the reasons whereby the delay of diagnosis seems to be longer in this subgroup compared to others. Nevertheless, the 'pseudo-sclerotic' variant has been associated with better clinical outcomes upon treatment (therapy of WD has been discussed in Case 11).

From the phenomenological standpoint, WD patients most commonly show irregular, sometimes asymmetric, and somewhat jerky tremor, which is thought to be dystonic in nature. Very rarely, a unilateral isolated rest tremor is seen. When rest tremor is present, it is almost invariably accompanied by postural and kinetic tremor, which is usually more severe than the rest tremor. It is, however, important to remark that WD can be very pleomorphic and, as Walshe stated, 'no two patients are ever the same, even in a sibship'.

Suggested Readings

Bandmann O, Weiss KH, Kaler SG. Wilson's disease and other neurological copper disorders. *Lancet Neurol.* 2015;14(1):103–13.

Lorincz MT. Neurologic Wilson's disease. *Ann N Y Acad Sci.* 2010;1184:173–87.

Walshe JM, Yealland M. Wilson's disease: the problem of delayed diagnosis. *J Neurol Neurosurg Psychiatry.* 1992;55:692–6.

Video 45.1

This patient has a postural tremor (left>right) when his arms are outstretched in front of him. However, his tremor changes pattern and increases in amplitude on his right arm with elbow flexed (wing position). There is also a bilateral action tremor as well as head titubation.

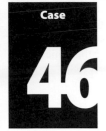

Roberto Erro and Kailash P. Bhatia

Case 46

Thalamic Tremor

Clinical History

This 82-year-old right-handed woman with medically treated hypertension and hypercholesterolemia abruptly developed tremor in her right upper limb, shortly after she was discharged from the A&E department for an episode of angina. The tremor was severe enough to interfere with her day-to-day activities. She mentioned that her tremor was most evident when holding objects, but could be present at times also at rest. She further mentioned that her balance was mildly affected and needed a walking stick for support. No further complaints were declared. Specifically, she did not feel that she had slowed down.

Examination

On examination, an irregular and fast tremor of her right hand, which was present at rest and on posture (see Video 46.1), with no kinetic tremor was found. The remaining neurological examination was unremarkable, apart from some enhancement of deep tendon reflexes of the right hemi-body. Specifically, there were no bradykinesia, rigidity, sensory or motor disturbances, and coordination and gait were tested normal.

General Remarks

In such a case, one obviously should consider PD in the differential diagnosis given the presence of a unilateral tremor with a rest component. However, as a general rule, one should first exclude structural lesions for any movement disorder that is strictly confined to one side of the body. In our patient, in fact there were other clinical clues, which were in keeping with this hypothesis. First, the acute development of tremor would fit in with a vascular etiology. Second, apart from tremor, deep tendon reflexes were found to be brisker on the same side, both in the upper and in the lower limb. Third, as

to the phenomenology, such a tremor was quite jerky and this is not the rule in PD. Finally, there were no other clinical features (i.e. bradykinesia) to suspect PD.

Investigations

Standard blood investigations were within normal limits. A brain MRI revealed a lateral-posterior stroke in the left thalamus (Figure 46.1), without involvement of the brainstem or the cerebellum, whereas a subsequent DaT-Scan was proven normal.

Special Remarks

Thalamic lesions including thalamic infarction or haemorrhage, infections, traumatic injury, and neoplasm typically result in a somatosensory syndrome in which some patients develop central neuropathic pain. However, rarely movement disorders can be also observed and include dystonia, tremor, and ballism. The occurrence of movement disorders after thalamic lesions can be as delayed as 4 years after an ischemic or haemorrhagic lesion of the posterior thalamus.

Isolated distal resting and intention tremor after thalamic infarction is exceedingly scarce and usually is associated with sensory disturbances or motor deficits. Tremor due to lateral-posterior thalamic lesions usually features a postural/intention component at 2–5 Hz, even though tremor at higher frequency has been described with posterior thalamic lesions. Furthermore, dystonic movements or abnormal posturing of the upper limb contralateral to the thalamic lesion can be seen.

The pathophysiological origin of thalamic tremor remains unknown. One possibility relies on the disruption between the posterior thalamus and mesencephalic and cerebellar area.

No specific treatment exists for this type of tremor and, as such, management should be pursued

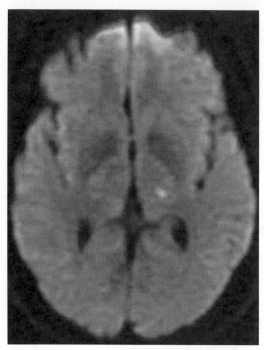

Figure 46.1 Axial DWI sequences showing a hyperintense signal corresponding to an ischemic stroke in the lateral-posterior region of the left thalamus.

empirically. However, deep brain stimulation, in particular stimulation of the internal globus pallidum, has recently been shown to improve both rest and intention components of tremor due to ischemic thalamic stroke.

Suggested Readings

Lee MS, Marsden CD. Movement disorders following lesions of the thalamus or subthalamic region. *Mov Disord*. 1994;9:493–507.

Miwa H, Hatori K, Kondo T, Imai H, Mizuno Y. Thalamic tremor: case reports and implications of the tremor-generating mechanism. *Neurology*. 1996;46:75–9.

Schmahmann JD. Vascular syndromes of the thalamus. *Stroke*. 2003;34:2264–78.

 Video 46.1

Irregular fast tremor of the right hand at rest and on posture is shown.

Shaking on Standing: Orthostatic Tremor

Roberto Erro and Kailash P. Bhatia

Clinical History

A 61-year-old woman, who has generally been in good health and with no family history for any neurological disorders, first came to our attention for a feeling of unsteadiness only when standing. Besides the unsteadiness, she mentioned that her leg would shake upon standing. Such an unsteadiness had started 4 years earlier and had progressively got worse, occasionally leading to a few falls. Holding onto something or walking would have allowed her to be stable. Tremor was apparently not present when sitting or lying down. More recently, she noted that her arms began shaking as well when holding some objects, but her arm tremor did not interfere with her day-to-day activities.

Examination

On examination, we found very little. In fact, she had an intermittent bilateral tremor of her arm on posture, which was not distractible or entrainable. When standing, nothing could be seen as to her legs, but a fine tremor could be appreciated upon touching her tights. Her neurological examination was otherwise normal.

General Remarks

The complaint of unsteadiness and shaking on standing that is relieved by sitting, walking, or holding onto something is very suggestive of OT. Yet, OT is an electrophysiological diagnosis and different OT-mimics can account for similar subjective feelings of unsteadiness/shaking on standing (Table 47.1). As such, an electrophysiological testing is mandatory and given the possible association of OT with PD, we would advocate that a DaT-Scan should be performed when there are additional signs such as bradykinesia or rigidity on examination.

Investigations

Electrophysiological recording of her tremor disclosed a high frequency tremor at about 15 Hz bilaterally in her legs, which was highly coherent between homologous muscle of the right and left leg. Moreover, a postural tremor at about 7.5 Hz could be detected in her arms. A brain MRI and a DaT-Scan were found to be normal. A diagnosis of primary OT was therefore made.

Special Remarks

Primary OT is largely considered sporadic, but very few familial cases have been reported. Women are predominantly affected (sex ratio: 2:1) and disease onset generally occurs in the sixth decade. Clinically, primary OT is associated with an intense and disabling sense of unsteadiness and a fear of falling, which stops when patients sit, walk, or use a support, and only a subset of patients specifically complains about shaking of their legs. Electrophysiologically, OT is characterized by a high frequency tremor (>13 Hz) of the legs that is highly synchronous between homologous leg muscles. Such features clearly differentiate OT from pseudo-OT (i.e. shaking on standing with tremor occurring at frequencies lower than 13 Hz) and orthostatic myoclonus (Table 47.1). Such a high-frequency tremor can be visible only as a fine-amplitude rippling of the leg muscles, palpable as a thrill, and heard by muscle auscultation as a thudding sound, similar to that of a distant helicopter. However, in the majority of patients with primary OT, an additional arm tremor at lower frequency develops. Yet, this lower-frequency postural arm tremor and similar lower-frequency components in the legs have been found to represent a subharmonic of the high-frequency OT observed in the legs and hence not generated independently.

Primary OT progress over time and response to treatment is highly variable between patients: some can respond to clonazepam or gabapentin, while trials with levetiracetam, primidone, and botulinum toxin injections into the tibialis anterior muscle have been proven unsuccessful. There have been a few patients

Table 47.1 Electrophsyiological Criteria of OT and Its Mimics

	Electro-physiological Features	Additional Features
Primary OT	(1) 13–18-Hz tremor of the legs upon standing (2) Tremor is highly coherent between homologous muscles of right and left leg	The majority of patients have 6–7-Hz postural tremor of the arms.
Secondary OT/OT-plus	13–18-Hz tremor of the legs upon standing, which can be (or not) highly coherent between homologous muscles of right and left leg	There is either clinical or imaging evidence of another neurological condition
Pseudo-OT	Tremor of the legs upon standing is below 13 Hz (with low coherence values between homologous muscles of right and left leg)	Almost invariably, associated with another neurological condition
Orthostatic Myoclonus	Irregular bursts of myoclonus of the legs upon standing. Frequency can range from 6 to 18 Hz and muscle bursts are usually 50 to 60 msec in duration	Can be isolated or associated with another neurological condition

Source: Modified from Erro et al., *Mov Disord Clin Pract*, 2014;1:173–9.

reported on who benefitted from thalamic DBS or spinal stimulation.

OT has been reported to be associated with a number of different conditions, hence generating the rational to classify patients into two broad rubrics: primary and secondary OT (or OT plus). PD is the most common condition associated with OT, and in some cases OT has been suggested to herald the onset of PD. As such, one might advocate a DaT-Scan in all patients presenting with OT, even in the absence of clear symptoms or signs suggestive of PD.

Suggested Readings

Erro R, Bhatia KP, Cordivari C. Shaking on standing: a critical review. *Mov Disord Clinic Pract*. 2014;1:173–9.

Ganos C, Maugest L, Apartis E, et al. The long-term outcome of orthostatic tremor. *J Neurol Neurosurg Psychiatry*. 2015. doi: 10.1136/jnnp-2014–309942.

Gerschlager W, Munchau A, Katzenschlager R, et al. Natural history and syndromic associations of orthostatic tremor: a review of 41 patients. *Mov Disord*. 2004;19:788–95.

Functional Palatal Tremor

Roberto Erro, Maria Stamelou, and Kailash P. Bhatia

Clinical History

This 66-year-old woman has a very long-standing history, spanning over 20 years, of abnormal semi-rhythmic movements of her palate, which are sometimes associated with ear clicks. Her symptoms started soon after a minor throat infection at the age of 43 years. The symptoms did not deteriorate significantly over the years, but in the past 5 or 6 years, she has also had occasional spasms of her lower face, which have been painful.

Examination

On examination (Video 48.1), the only abnormality that could be detected was a semi-rhythmic activity of her palate and posterior tongue at about 2.5 Hz, which was associated with an audible click. Such a tremor was present with her mouth closed or wide open, but not when she was speaking. Moreover, the tremor could be stopped when she was asked to tap with her right hand, regardless of the frequency of the tapping.

Investigations and Diagnosis

A brain MRI was proven normal. Specifically, no lesions or abnormalities could be seen in the Guillain–Mollaret triangle. A sub-therapeutic dosage of botulinum toxin was injected into the posterior palatal wall and a complete resolution of the tremor was observed within few minutes, suggestive of a placebo response. By history, examination and complete resolution after placebo, this patient fulfilled the criteria for the definitive diagnosis of functional (psychogenic) palatal tremor.

Remarks

PT (or palatal myoclonus) is characterized by rhythmic movements of the soft palate, usually at a frequency ranging from 0.5 to 3 Hz. PT is classically classified as essential (or primary or isolated) when PT (with or without ear clicks) is the only feature and all investigations are normal, and as symptomatic (or secondary) when PT is owing to, most commonly, structural lesions in the Guillain–Mollaret triangle. The latter, also known as the dentato-rubro-olivary tract, has in fact three interconnected nodes: the red nucleus via the central tegmental tract projects to the inferior olivary nucleus that, via the inferior cerebellar peduncle, projects to the contralateral dentate nucleus and back to the red nucleus via the superior cerebellar peduncle. Symptomatic PT is associated with hypertrophic olivary degeneration, a rare form of transsynaptic degeneration causing hypertrophy (which is a unique phenomenon in the central nervous system) of the inferior olives and is detectable as hyperintensity of the inferior olives on MRI. However, secondary PT has also been rarely reported to be associated with genetic/degenerative conditions, including Alexander disease, neuroferritinopathy, or as part of PAPT syndrome.

The pathophysiology of essential PT is instead elusive and recent large-series appraisal has documented that a vast majority of such cases could be functional (psychogenic) in nature. The patient presented here shared with published series on FMD a number of commonalities, including gender, presence of a minor physical event precipitating the movement disorder, and associated functional symptoms/signs (e.g. painful spasms of the lower face). Moreover, there were on examination positive findings supportive of a functional PT, such as the distractibility of the PT when performing different motor tasks. It is likely that these maneuvers were not performed in old series on PT, therefore accounting for the under-recognition of some of the functional PT cases. The importance of the diagnosis of FMD has crucial implications in terms of management, since it has been demonstrated that failure (and delay) in providing a correct diagnosis and appropriate treatments are indicators of poor recovery.

Suggested Readings

Deuschl G, Wilms H. Clinical spectrum and physiology of palatal tremor. *Mov Disord*. 2002;17(Suppl 2):S63–6.

Stamelou M, Saifee TA, Edwards MJ, Bhatia KP. Psychogenic palatal tremor may be under recognized: reappraisal of a large series of cases. *Mov Disord*. 2012;27(9):1164–8.

Zadikoff C, Lang AE, Klein C. The 'essentials' of essential palatal tremor: a reappraisal of the nosology. *Brain*. 2006;129(Pt 4):832–40.

Video 48.1

Palatal tremor which completely stops when the patient is asked to tap with her fingers.

Case

49

Dystonic Tremor and Progressive Ataxia: SCA12

Christos Ganos and Kailash P. Bhatia

Clinical History

A woman of Indian origin presented to our clinic at the age of 36 with a 5-year-long history of a tremulous disorder that has affected her neck/head, face, voice, and arms. The first symptom, a right-arm action tremor appeared post-partum at the age of 31. Over the ensuing years, her left arm and the craniocervical region also became tremulous. Initially, she reported some benefit after the intake of small amounts of alcohol. There were no further symptoms at the time. There was a positive family history. The patient's father, who resided in India, was reported to suffer from tremor of the head and had, in fact, been receiving botulinum toxin injections with some improvement. Further, a paternal uncle also appeared to be affected by tremulous movements of the hands and head. The patient, who was initially diagnosed with ET, was then referred to our department for further evaluation and treatment.

Examination

At the age of 36, oculomotor examination was normal. There was an irregular head tremor with improvement on certain head positions, which also affected the face (eyebrows/mouth), tongue, and jaw. There was adductor dysphonia. She had clear torticollis and laterocollis. There was a jerky asymmetric kinetic arm tremor (right>left) with mild dystonic hand posturing on both sides (see Video 49.1). There was no intention tremor. Strength and muscle tone examination, as well as reflexes, were unrevealing. There were no sensory abnormalities. There was no bradykinesia. Heel-to-shin testing, stance and gait, including tandem, were normal. Neuropsychiatric assessment was unrevealing.

General Remarks

This lady, a young adult, initially developed a tremulous disorder affecting her right arm, which within a period of 5 years spread to affect her other arm, as well as the craniocervical area. She also manifested adductor

dysphonia. Probably due to the initially seemingly isolated presentation of the action tremor of one, and then both arms, in the presence of some alcohol responsiveness and a positive family history this patient was diagnosed with essential tremor. However, the presentation of clear dystonic symptoms argues against this diagnosis and alongside other tremor characteristics, such as tremor distribution in areas also affected by dystonic symptoms, tremor irregularity and improvement of tremor on certain head positions the diagnosis of a dystonic tremor was rendered most likely. Among the conditions that can present with prominent dystonic upper limb and head tremor, including voice tremor and adductor dysphonia in the absence of further symptoms, and in the presence of positive family history, the diagnosis of a primary (or according to the new dystonia classification, an isolated, inherited) dystonic condition should be considered. Within this spectrum of conditions, *Anoctamin-3* gene mutations (*ANO3*; DYT24) have been recently recognized to present with a predominant tremulous dystonic phenotype of craniocervical (including laryngeal) and upper limb muscles. However, no *ANO3* mutations have been reported yet in patients of Indian origin. On the contrary, autosomal-dominant SCA may also present with a combination of (usually titubatory) head and upper limb tremor, and further symptoms, including dystonia, in the absence of prominent ataxia, particularly during the first years of illness in younger patients. Among these disorders, pathological CAG repeat expansions of the *PPP2R2B* (SCA12) have been commonly associated with prominent action tremor of hands and head presenting in the 4th life decade and in patients of Indian descent.

Investigations and Diagnosis

Routine laboratory blood work, including serum copper/ceruloplasmin, was normal. A brain MRI revealed mild generalized volume loss. Surface electromyography and accelerometry with electrodes placed on the right sternocleidomastoid, biceps, extensor carpi radialis, and first dorsal interossei muscles showed a 4-Hz tremor of head and arms with variable amplitude, more pronounced during posture and kinesis. Superimposed jerks in her arms with burst duration more than 100 ms and no clear muscular progression, and also longer bursts, up to 3–4 seconds, consistent with slow dystonic movements were noted.

Given the aforementioned differential diagnosis and considering the patient's Indian origin, testing for CAG repeat length in the *PPP2R2B* gene was performed. A pathological repeat expansion in one allele was found (52/11 repeats), and the diagnosis of SCA12 was made. It should be noted that, at the age of 38 (Video 49.1), the patient further developed progressive balance difficulties. Neurological examination revealed the additional presence of cerebellar ataxia, in line with the aforementioned genetic diagnosis.

Special Remarks

Autosomal-dominant inherited SCAs comprise an expanding group of heterogeneous disorders with the hallmark feature of cerebellar degeneration. Although in most SCAs there is phenotypic overlap, certain clinical signs cluster around particular SCA subtypes. In this regard, SCA12, a rather rare SCA subtype, has been associated with prominent action tremor of the arms and head at symptom onset. This syndromic association is, in fact, so prominent that it has prompted screening study for the presence of *PPP2R2B* gene CAG repeat expansions in familial cases diagnosed with ET, albeit with negative results. Mean age of symptom onset is in the 4th life decade. Although dystonic symptoms have been described in some SCA12 cases (e.g. 'axial' dystonia, laterocollis, or foot dystonia), predominant craniocervical and laryngeal involvement have not been reported beyond this case. Also, no previous report has elaborated on

the nature of tremor being dystonic in SCA12, as in the presented case. Brain MRI usually demonstrates mild generalized supra- and/or cerebellar atrophy. Although initially described in an American pedigree of German descent, the vast majority of identified families are of Indian origin. The CAG length range for normal alleles is between 4 and 32 triplets, but this may expand as more individuals undergo testing. On the contrary, it is still unclear what the shortest pathogenic repeat range and repeat length for complete penetrance are. Recent evidence, however, suggests that triplet expansions beyond 46 repeats should be considered pathogenic.

Suggested Readings

Holmes SE, O'Hearn EE, McInnis MG, et al. Expansion of a novel CAG trinucleotide repeat in the 50 region of PPP2R2B is associated with SCA12. *Nat Genet.* 1999;23:391–2.

Srivastava AK, Choudhry S, Gopinath MS, et al. Molecular and clinical correlation in five Indian families with spinocerebellar ataxia 12. *Ann Neurol.* 2001;50:796–800.

Stamelou M, Charlesworth G, Cordivari C, et al. The phenotypic spectrum of DYT24 due to ANO3 mutations. *Mov Disord.* 2014;29:928–34.

Video 49.1

This patient has a mild torticollis and laterocollis with associated head tremor at about 4 Hz. Irregular jaw and lip tremor during neck extension is seen. She has adductor-type dystonic voice tremor and an irregular, jerky tongue tremor as well as facial (eyebrow/perioral) tremor. Jerky dystonic arm tremor and dystonic hand posturing (right>left) is seen. In addition, she has bilateral intention tremor, decomposition of movement on finger–nose test, and a megalographic dysgraphia.

Case

50

Bilateral Holmes Tremor in MS

Roberto Erro and Kailash P. Bhatia

Clinical History and Examination

A 34-year-old woman diagnosed with secondary progressive MS since the age of 21 years was admitted into the hospital for the development of a severe tremor of her upper limbs.

On examination (see Video 50.1), it was revealed that she had a coarse tremor of her upper limbs at rest, augmented with posture and action. Besides her tremor, she had dysarthria and dysphagia, which required the placement of a feeding tube. Moreover, she had broken smooth pursuits, proximal weakness in the lower limbs, along with spasticity, brisk deep tendon reflexes, and bilateral positive Babinski's sign. The Expanded Disability Status Scale was 8.0.

Investigations

A brain MRI showed diffuse demyelinated plaques both in the supratentorial and infratentorial areas. In particular, two large plaques were noted in the pons and mesencephalon, thus supporting a diagnosis of Holmes tremor in the context of MS.

Remarks

The exact prevalence of tremor in the MS population is not entirely known, with estimates ranging from 25 and 60 per cent of patients. The two most prevalent tremor forms in MS are postural tremor and intention tremor, due to cerebellar dysfunction, while Holmes tremor is considered to be rare, with one study failing to show one single case among 100 MS patients.

First described by Gordon Holmes in 1904, Holmes tremor is by definition a combination of rest, action, and postural tremor, with a frequency ranging from 3 to 5 Hz, and associated with midbrain lesions in the vicinity of the red nucleus (thereby also referred to as 'rubral' tremor). In the series described by Holmes, tremor occurred at rest, similar to the classical rest tremor seen in PD, and on posture and was worse on movement, particularly when approaching the target.

It consists of irregular flexion and extension of the fingers with rotation at the wrist and elbow, and is usually unilateral. Holmes tremor may arise from various underlying structural disorders, including multiple sclerosis, stroke, head trauma, tumors, and infections. There may be a variable delay of 2 weeks to 2 years between the precipitating event and the initial appearance of tremor. Although the original definition of Holmes tremor requires the presence of all three tremor components, a few patients have been described with only minimal or no postural tremor. The subsequent criteria have therefore been suggested to define Holmes tremor: (1) the presence of a rest and action tremor, with or without a postural component, often irregular and less rhythmic than other types of tremor; (2) a slow frequency, usually under 4.5 Hz; and (3) if the tremor is secondary to an identifiable lesion, there is a variable delay before the onset of tremor, usually amounting to months.

Holmes tremor has been reported to occur as a consequence of a lesion damaging both the ascending dopaminergic pathways from substantia nigra to striatum (producing the 'parkinsonian' rest tremor) and the cerebellothalamic/cerebelloolivary systems. Most of the patients with Holmes tremor have other signs of midbrain damage, including oculomotor abnormalities and hemiparesis.

Described in general, it is poorly responsive to treatment. However, as the dopaminergic system is involved in most cases, treatment with levodopa should be attempted even though dyskinesias have been reported to occur in some cases. Drugs used for the treatment of ET may also be effective, and thalamic DBS has proven beneficial. Yet, there is the problem that additional ataxia (which often occurs in patients with MS) is not improved and may be worsened. Moreover, usually there is a strong correlation between presence of tremor in MS and higher disability, making it difficult to establish a realistic view of the outcome.

Suggested Readings

Alusi SH, Worthington J, Glickman S, Bain PG. A study of tremor in multiple sclerosis. *Brain*. 2001;124:720–30.

Deuschl G, Wilms H, Krack P, Würker M, Heiss WD. Function of the cerebellum in Parkinsonian rest tremor and Holmes' tremor. *Ann Neurol*. 1999;46:126–8.

Rinker JR 2nd, Salter AR, Walker H, et al. Prevalence and characteristics of tremor in the NARCOMS multiple sclerosis registry: a cross-sectional survey. *BMJ Open*. 2015;5:e006714.

Video 50.1

A bilateral rest, postural, and action tremor with low frequency and high amplitude is seen.

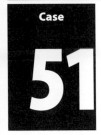

Case

51

Primary Writing Tremor

Roberto Erro and Kailash P. Bhatia

Clinical History

This is a 73-year-old right-handed man of Indian origin, who had been in general good health, not requiring any medications on long-term basis. Over the past 5 years, he has had mildly progressive difficulties featuring shaking of his right hand at certain angles, only upon writing. He mentioned that this was particularly obvious when he had to perform anticlockwise movement as part of his signature. His general practitioner tried him on anti-cholinergics and propranolol, both of which were proven unhelpful. His tremor was not improved by alcohol and did not affect any other day-to-day activities. There were no additional complaints. As to his family history, his parents were not blood relatives and had not suffered from any neurologic disorders, but his older brother (aged 76) had developed tremor since the age of 72 years, while his niece (aged 43) had developed abnormal posturing of her right hand, but no tremor, since her late twenties.

Examination

On examination (see Video 51.1), we found that he had a tremor of his right arm while he was writing, while no tremor could be seen at rest or on posture. Moreover, there was no tremor when he was asked to perform other movements, for instance, pouring some water from one glass into another. There was a doubtful dystonic posturing of his fingers whilst keeping his arms outstretched. The remaining neurological examination was normal.

Investigations and Diagnosis

Standard biochemical investigations as well as a brain MRI were entirely normal. Given the possible family history for dystonia, he was tested for mutations in the *TOR1A* gene (responsible for DYT1, cf. Table 16.1), but found to be negative. He was eventually diagnosed with PWT.

Remarks

PWT is a rare tremor syndrome that occurs with writing, the pathophysiology of which is still unknown. Patients with PWT have been sub-classified as having either a task-induced tremor (depending on whether tremor appeared only during writing) or positionally sensitive tremor (i.e. when tremor occurs whilst writing and adopting the hand position used in writing). The latter sub-group would imply that PWT is a dystonic condition, where the tremor occurs only when adopting some particular postures associated with writing. However, there has been debate about this entity since it has been construed to be also a form of ET by some authors. Our case supports the view that PWT could be dystonic in nature (despite there was no overt dystonia on examination), given the presence of one affected subject in this family with clear dystonia and no tremor. Complicating this issue, there has been one family reported on with PWT, ET, and writer's cramp, suggesting some overlap between these conditions. However, it would be unwise to consider ET in our patient, given the very late onset of his symptoms and the asymmetry of his tremor. Moreover, his family history strongly argues for dystonia as the unifying theme of this autosomal dominant disorder with marked clinical heterogeneity.

Suggested Readings

Bain PG, Findley LJ, Britton TC, et al. Primary writing tremor. *Brain*. 1995;118:1461–72.

Cohen LG, Hallett M, Sudarsky L. A single family with writer's cramp, essential tremor, and primary writing tremor. *Mov Disord*. 1987;2:109–16.

Pita Lobo P, Quattrocchi G, Jutras MF, et al. Primary writing tremor and writer's cramp: two faces of a same coin? *Mov Disord*. 2013;28:1306–7.

Rothwell JC, Traub MM, Marsden CD. Primary writing tremor. *J Neurol Neurosurg Psychiatry*. 1979;42:1106–14.

Video 51.1

There is a tremor of his right arm only on writing, while no tremor can be seen at rest, on posture, or on action.

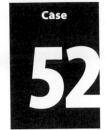

A Case of Myoclonus-Dystonia

Roberto Erro, Maria Stamelou, and Kailash P. Bhatia

Clinical History

This 37-year-old right-handed man with no family history was referred for a very long-standing history of depression and jerks, which had recently worsened following bereavement in the family. He had a normal birth and milestones. At the age of 4, he was noted to have jerks in the legs, which subsequently spread to his arms. This left him with problems in writing at school. Around the same time, he was also noted to have mood swings, and his school performance declined. After an initial worsening, he has been stable for a while, but jerks were still quite violent so that he broke his upper teeth by trying to eat with a fork. He could also fall over because of the leg jerks. He denied any benefit from alcohol on his jerks.

Examination

On examination (see Video 52.1), eye movements and cranial nerves were found to be normal. He had clear retrocollic 'shock-like' as well as less brusque proximal limb jerks. The jerks were not stimulus sensitive. Gait was impaired because of his leg jerks, with some tandem walking difficulties. Furthermore, he had a slight torticollis to the right with tilting to the left and left shoulder elevation, whereas the remaining neurological examination was normal.

General Remarks

The combination of myoclonic jerks with such a body distribution (in the neck and proximally in the limbs) and subtle dystonia suggests the diagnosis of myoclonus-dystonia, despite the absence of a positive family history for myoclonus and/or dystonia as well as the absence of alcohol responsiveness. The psychiatric profile in our patient would also be in keeping with such a diagnosis. The somatic localization would instead be against other myoclonic conditions, including FCMTE, where jerks are most localized distally in the limbs and can resemble a tremor (cf. Case 58).

Investigations and Diagnosis

Standard blood investigations and a brain MRI were normal. Electrophysiological testing revealed the jerks to be of relatively short duration (around 150 msec) and jerk-locked averaging did not show any cortical correlates. Genetic testing for the ε-sarcoglycan gene (*SGCE*) was pursued and it was revealed that he was a carrier of the missense c.T7774A mutation, thus confirming a diagnosis of DYT11(cf. Table 16.1).

Special Remarks

Classically, the term 'myoclonus-dystonia' was used to describe an autosomal dominant entity featuring dystonia and myoclonus responsive to alcohol, which has been subsequently proven to be due to *SGCE* mutations in the majority of patients (up to 50 per cent of familial cases). Although, by definition, both myoclonus and dystonia should be present, it has become clear that dystonia might be subtle and the clinical picture dominated by myoclonus. This is confirmed by the high inter-family clinical variability with affected subjects who can exhibit either lightning myoclonic jerks or dystonia, or both. Sometimes alcohol responsiveness might be absent as in our case. The myoclonic jerks are brief, lightning-like, and generally limited to the upper body. Dystonia is present in about half of the cases in the form of cervical dystonia or writer's cramp without tendency to the generalization. The onset is in childhood or early adolescence and there is a usually a positive family history, although the penetrance of this disorder is incomplete. There is evidence for maternal imprinting, with symptomatic carriers usually inheriting the mutation from the father. Large *SGCE* deletions are associated with more complex phenotypes due to haploinsufficiency of adjacent genes and carriers might manifest with short stature, microcephaly, sensorineural hearing loss, dysmorphic features, and psychomotor delay.

As mentioned earlier, a significant proportion of patients carrying a *SGCE* mutation manifest with isolated myoclonus and electrophysiological testing can be hence useful for the differential diagnosis with other myoclonic disorders. *SGCE* carriers show in fact a homogeneous electrophysiologic pattern of myoclonus of subcortical origin with short jerks (25–250 msec) with no features of cortical hyperexcitability (namely, no abnormal C-reflex response and no short-latency premyoclonic potential on back-averaging). In the absence of genetic testing, electrophysiology can be of great value in differentiating cortical from subcortical myoclonus to lead treatment choice. In fact, myoclonus-dystonia patients are likely to respond to clonazepam, while antiepileptics are of little utility.

Worth noting, a proportion of patients with myoclonus-dystonia do not carry *SGCE* mutations, suggesting genetic variability. Recently, *KCTD17* mutations have been reported to cause myoclonus-dystonia (cf. Table 16.1) and should be hence considered in the differential diagnosis. Differently from *SCGE* carriers, in patients with *KCTD17* mutations dystonia seems to dominate the clinical picture with a tendency of progression to other sites (including larynx with speech involvement), a course that is unusual for *SGCE*-related myoclonus-dystonia. Moreover, myoclonus, despite being the presenting symptom in most of *KCTD17* cases, is overall mild and not as disabling as in *SGCE*-mutated subjects.

Suggested Readings

Nardocci N. Myoclonus-dystonia syndrome. *Handb Clin Neurol.* 2011;100:563–75.

Quinn NP. Essential myoclonus and myoclonic dystonia. *Mov Disord.* 1996;11:119–24.

Roze E, Apartis E, Clot F et al. Myoclonus-dystonia: clinical and electrophysiologic pattern related to SGCE mutations. *Neurology.* 2008;70:1010–16.

Video 52.1

Generalized myoclonus is shown, with clear retrocollic 'shock-like' as well as less brusque proximal limb jerks. The jerks are not stimulus sensitive. He also has a slight torticollis to the right.

Case

53

Progressive Myoclonic Ataxia and Unverricht-Lundborg Disease

Roberto Erro, Bettina Balint, and Kailash P. Bhatia

Clinical History

This 60-year-old lady with no family history for any neurological disorder was admitted at the age of 45 years for the worsening of her symptoms, which began at the age of 12, when she started having myoclonic seizures. Her seizures were well controlled with a combination of anti-epileptics, but she progressively developed jerks of her face, voice, and limbs. Her jerks were most evident on action. She also complained about being progressively unsteady, and a few falls occurred.

Examination

On examination, it was found that she had square wave jerks, but otherwise her ocular movements were normal. There were spontaneous myoclonic jerks involving her head and trunk, as well as jerks of the upper limbs when outstretched and of her legs when walking. She also had bilateral upper limb ataxia on the finger–nose test, and her gait was broad based. The remaining neurological examination was normal.

General Remarks

The combination of progressive myoclonus and ataxia amounts to what has been referred to as PMA, Ramsay Hunt syndrome or dyssynergia cerebellaris myoclonica. There is a considerable overlap with the group of PME, and the differential diagnosis and further investigations should be guided by the presence of associated features, particularly by the presence or absence of cognitive decline (Table 53.1). Additional clinical clues can come from signs like visual disturbance, hepatosplenomegaly, or skeletal deformities, whereas basic laboratory parameters (e.g. CK, renal profile) may provide complementary information. The significance of electrophysiological investigations (SSEP, EMG with back averaging, C-Reflex, EEG) lies in establishing the origin of myoclonus (cortical vs. subcortical). Determination of the pattern of EEG abnormalities or myopathic findings may also be helpful.

Investigations and Diagnosis

Standard biochemical investigations were normal. An EEG disclosed generalized spike and wave discharges. Jerks-locked back-averaging EEG disclosed enlarged SSEPs ("giant SSEP") and a cortical correlate to the jerks on back averaging. Duodenal and muscle biopsy were normal. A formal neuropsychometry was performed and did not disclose any deficits, apart from a mild executive dysfunction.

PCR analysis flanking the dodecamer repeat sequence in the *CSTB* gene detected two expanded fragments of approximately 488 and 500 bp, representing alleles of 37 and 38 dodecamer repeats, thus confirming the diagnosis of ULD.

Special Remarks

ULD is an autosomal recessively inherited disorder, caused by mutations in the *CSTB* (cystatin B) gene, and represents the most common cause of PME. Onset of ULD is usually between 6 and 16 years. The symptoms at onset can be either myoclonic jerks (in more than half of the patients) and/or generalized tonic–clonic seizures. The myoclonic jerks are action-induced and often stimulus-sensitive, and may be provoked by light, physical exertion, noise, and stress. Jerks can generalize to a series of myoclonic seizures or even to a status myoclonicus. Epileptic seizures are not very frequent, but possible, in the very early stages of the disease. Yet, they often increase in frequency during the following 3–7 years, to entirely cease with appropriate anticpileptic treatments. Myoclonic jerks are instead often disabling and resistant to therapy. Usually some years after the onset, ataxia, intentional tremor, and dysarthria develop. Cognition is generally preserved, but affected subjects can show emotional liability and depression. The disease is inevitably progressive and about one-third of the patients become severely incapacitated and/or wheelchair bound.

Table 53.1 Differential Diagnosis of Mycolonus-Ataxia Syndromes

Condition	Gene(s)	Inheritance	Clinical Clues/Notes
With no or very mild cognitive impairment			
Unverricht–Lundborg (Baltic myoclonus)	CSTB	AR	Photosensitivity and photoparoxysmal response on EEG
Progressive myoclonus epilepsy-ataxia syndrome	PRICKLE1	AR	Impaired upgaze
Action myoclonus-renal failure syndrome	SCARB2	AR	Renal failure not obligatory
North sea myoclonus	GOSR2	AR	Arreflexia, scoliosis
Myoclonus epilepsy and ataxia due to potassium channel mutation (MEAK)	KCNC1	AD	–
SCA14	PRKCG	AD	Spasticity, dystonia
Coeliac disease	N/A	N/A	Presence of gliadin / tissue transglutaminase antibodies; diarrhea
Ataxia teleangiectasia	ATM	AR	Oculomotor apraxia, teleangiectasias
With or without cognitive impairment			
Dentato-rubro-pallido-luysian atrophy (DRPLA)	ATN1	AD	Most common in the Japanese population
Mitochondrial disorders, e.g. MERRF	MTTK, MTTL1, MTTH, MTTS1, MTTS2, MTTF	Maternal	Short stature, deafness, myopathy
With dementia			
Lafora disease	EPM2A or NHLRC1	AR	Occipital seizures
Neuronal ceroid lipofuscinosis	CLN1-10	AR/AD	Visual disturbance, extrapyramidal symptoms
Sialidosis	NEU1 or PPBG	AR	Visual disturbance, cherry red spot, skeletal dysplasia, hepatomegaly
Prion disease	PRNP	AD or sporadic	Rapid disease progression
Niemann-Pick C	NPC1, NPC2	AR	Hepatosplenomegaly, vertical supranuclear gaze palsy
Gaucher Type III	GBA	AR	Hepatosplenomegaly, horizontal supranuclear gaze palsy

Abb.: AR: Autosomal recessive; AD: Autosomal dominant; N/A: not applicable.

Suggested Readings

Chew NK, Mir P, Edwards MJ, et al. The natural history of Unverricht-Lundborg disease: a report of eight genetically proven cases. *Mov Disord*. 2008;23:107–13.

Kälviäinen R, Khyuppenen J, Koskenkorva P, Eriksson K, Vanninen R, Mervaala E. Clinical picture of EPM1-Unverricht-Lundborg disease. *Epilepsia*. 2008;49:549–56.

North Sea Myoclonus Due to *GOSR2* Mutations

Bettina Balint and Kailash P. Bhatia

Clinical History

During her second year of life, this patient was noted to be mildly unsteady with occasional falls. In her childhood, she had a few episodes of worsening of these symptoms, triggered by infections and fever, and one episode of severe encephalopathy at age 3. Between these episodes she had excellent recoveries and attended a normal school till age 11. Subsequently she developed generalized jerks, mainly on action, and later on epilepsy around age 14. Whereas, aged 16, she was independent and able to feed herself (even though drinking with a straw), write, knit, and play the piano, her symptoms got progressively worse after age 17. In her twenties she started using the wheelchair for longer distances, and around age 30 she became wheelchair-bound and dependent for the basic activities of daily living. Her cognitive function has always been good, although a mild decline was noted on repeated formal testing. She has also developed urinary incontinence requiring treatment with antimuscarinic drugs. Currently, she is 61 years old and lives at a residential care facility. There is no significant family history and no consanguinity.

Examination

On examination (Video 54.1), she showed frequent and violent action and stimulus sensitive myoclonus mainly affecting her upper limbs, neck, and face. Spontaneous myoclonus was present to a lesser extent. Her speech was very slurred and interrupted by the myoclonus. Her eye movements featured broken pursuit and gaze-evoked nystagmus. There was marked limb dysmetria, and some dystonic posturing of both hands and the neck. She additionally had a scoliosis and arreflexia. Bedside cognitive examination did not reveal gross deficits.

General Remarks

This patient presented in her infancy with a progressive syndrome featuring gait ataxia, myoclonus, and epilepsy. Cerebellar ataxia and myoclonus are the hallmark features of PMA. While the differential diagnosis in such cases is quite broad (cf. Case 53 and Table 53.1), there were a few clinical clues allowing narrowing down the possible aetiologies responsible for the clinical syndrome of the above patient. In her case one would notice the fairly benign course of the disease with preserved cognition on one hand, and the clinical signs of scoliosis and arreflexia on the other hand. On clinical grounds only, this combination would already suggest a diagnosis of 'North Sea myoclonus'.

Investigations and Diagnosis

A variety of blood tests including serum CK were normal, while her brain imaging showed generalized but mild atrophy. Her EEG featured a slowed background, generalized epileptiform transients, and photo-paroxysmal response. On electrophysiology, brief episodes of loss of tone were detectable as well as positive jerks of short duration and a latency of spread among different muscles compatible with a pyramidal progression, in keeping with cortical myoclonus. Back-averaging was not possible due to the high frequency of the jerks.

On genetic testing of *GOSR2*, she was found to be compound heterozygous for the c.430G>T (p.G144W) mutation and a novel deletion c.491_493delAGA (p.K164del), thus confirming the diagnosis of North Sea myoclonus.

Special Remarks

North Sea myoclonus is an autosomal recessive disorder due to mutations of *GOSR2*, encoding the Golgi SNAP receptor complex 2, which holds a role in protein transport from the endoplasmic reticulum and into the Golgi apparatus. The name relates to the fact that the birthplaces of all patients harbouring the c.430G>T (p.Gly144Trp) mutation, or their ancestors, cluster around the North Sea. Within the group of PME/PMA (cf. Table 34.1), North Sea myoclonus has a comparatively benign disease course and a fairly homogenous presentation. Most of the cases feature early onset of ataxia (around 2 years of age) which stands in contrast to the most common of these syndromes (e.g. ULD). Myoclonic seizures usually occur around age 6–7. Scoliosis develops typically during adolescence, but other skeletal deformities like syndactyly or *pes cavus* can also be observed. Often there are episodes of worsening associated with febrile illness. The disease follows a relentless course and patients become wheelchair-bound, and eventually bedridden, often requiring PEG tubes due to dysphagia. Death occurs in the second or third decade due to aspiration pneumonia, respiratory compromise, or status epilepticus. The EEG typically displays generalized spike and wave discharges with a posterior predominance and photosensitivity. Brain MRI may be normal, or show cerebellar or global atrophy. North Sea myoclonus was described only recently, and it is possible that the phenotypic and genotypic spectrum will expand. Our patient might be a good example of that, since she had a more benign disease course and no raised CK levels as well as one novel *GOSR2* mutation (c.491_493delAGA; p.K164del).

Suggested Readings

Boissé Lomax L, Bayly MA, Hjalgrim H, et al. 'North Sea' progressive myoclonus epilepsy: phenotype of subjects with GOSR2 mutation. *Brain*. 2013;136:1146–54.

Corbett MA, Schwake M, Bahlo M, et al. A mutation in the Golgi Qb-SNARE gene GOSR2 causes progressive myoclonus epilepsy with early ataxia. *Am J Hum Genet*. 2011;88:657–63.

van Egmond ME, Verschuuren-Bemelmans CC, Nibbeling EA, et al. Ramsay Hunt syndrome: clinical characterization of progressive myoclonus ataxia caused by GOSR2 mutation. *Mov Disord*. 2014;29:139–43.

Video 54.1

The video shows the patient at age 55. She is confined to the wheelchair. There are generalized myoclonic jerks (affecting face, neck, arms, and to a lesser degree legs), which become much more pronounced on action or even with visual stimuli. For example, during smooth pursuit eye movements, the jerks affecting her neck become quite violent. There is mild end-gaze nystagmus. When she is holding her arms outstretched, positive and negative myoclonus impedes her holding the arms still and interferes with testing for dysmetria. Myoclonus can be elicited by light touch. Other features comprise abolished deep tendon reflexes and scoliosis.

55

Progressive Myoclonic Ataxia and Coeliac Disease

Roberto Erro and Kailash P. Bhatia

Clinical History

This 49-year-old right-handed man came to us because of a 4-year history of tremor and balance difficulties. He had been generally in good health, apart from a diagnosis of coeliac disease that had been made 12 years earlier and for which he has been on a non-strict gluten-free diet since then. At 45 years of age, he had a two-month bout of diarrhea and stomach cramps. Shortly after the resolution of the gastrointestinal problems, he started noticing a tremor of his right hand and subsequently of his left hand. Moreover, he mentioned that he developed jerks, which were more apparent in his lower rather than his upper limbs. For example, he was having great difficulty putting his sock on because his feet would jump. He further complained about his balance, which developed around a year after the diarrhoea. This also worsened over time and represented the main complaint when he came to see us.

Examination

On examination (see Video 55.1), eye movements and cranial nerves were found to be normal. He had some facial twitches involving the upper part of his face. There were spontaneous and stimulus-sensitive jerks of his upper limbs when outstretched. Moreover, sudden loss of tone in his arms could be observed. Action-induced jerks were also seen in his legs. There was a mild dysmetria on the finger-nose test and he had an ataxic gait. Apart from brisk tendon reflexes, the remaining neurological examination was normal. Particularly, there was no evidence of peripheral sensory neuropathy.

General Remarks

The combination of progressive cerebellar signs and myoclonus, which on clinical ground was claimed to be cortical in origin mainly because of the stimulus-sensitiveness, amounts to what has been referred to as PMA, the Ramsay Hunt syndrome or dyssynergia cerebellaris myoclonica (cf. Cases 53 and 54). A number of pathological causes for this syndrome is now recognized (cf. Table 53.1) and therefore the diagnostic work-up should be pursued accordingly. However, there were a number of clinical features pointing towards one particular diagnosis. The age at onset would not fit with many of the disorders known to cause the Ramsay Hunt syndrome including ULD, Lafora disease, sialidosis, and neuronal ceroid lipofuscinosis. Moreover, our patient had been diagnosed with coeliac disease, and the latter has indeed been associated with the Ramsay Hunt syndrome. Other progressive conditions that can present with a combination of ataxia and myoclonus include DRPLA and MERRF.

Investigations and Diagnosis

Standard blood investigations were all normal, apart from a high titer of anti-transglutaminase antibodies (36.5 U/mL). A brain MRI was grossly normal, apart from some cerebellar atrophy. The electrophysiological recording of his left upper limb jerks was in keeping with a cortical origin of the myoclonus. Specifically, jerks were of short duration (between 25 and 50 msec) and had a definite pyramidal pattern of activation. Moreover, brief episodes of loss of tone were detectable consistent with negative myoclonus. Standard EEG was instead normal. Genetic screening for the *cystatin B*, *EPM2A*, and *DRPLA* genes and common mitochondrial mutations were negative. Moreover, muscle biopsy and ocular assessment were both normal. Altogether, these findings were in keeping with coeliac disease being the most likely etiology for the syndrome.

Special Remarks

There have been several cases reported in the literature with coeliac disease and PMA, suggesting a causal association between them. Nevertheless, the exact pathophysiological mechanisms of such an association are not entirely clear. In fact, despite improvement of the gastrointestinal symptoms on a gluten-free diet, the neurological syndrome usually shows steady progression, indicating that the latter is not due to malabsorption. Indeed, no specific deficiencies were found that could account for the progressive myoclonic ataxia in any of the patients reported so far. Furthermore, it remains to be determined why only a subset of patients with coeliac disease, which is fairly common in the general population, would develop such a neurological syndrome.

Post-mortem examination of the brain has been reported to show selective symmetrical atrophy of the cerebellar hemispheres with Purkinje cell loss and Bergmann astrocytosis, whereas cerebral hemispheres and brainstem were preserved.

As far as therapy is concerned, immunotherapy has not been found to be beneficial, and strict adherence to a gluten-free diet does not seem to prevent progression of the neurological syndrome. Symptomatic treatment of the myoclonus can be helpful in some cases.

Suggested Readings

Bhatia KP, Brown P, Gregory R, et al. Progressive myoclonic ataxia associated with coeliac disease. The myoclonus is of cortical origin, but the pathology is in the cerebellum. *Brain*. 1995;118:1087–93.

Ganos C, Kassavetis P, Erro R, Edwards MJ, Rothwell J, Bhatia KP. The role of the cerebellum in the pathogenesis of cortical myoclonus. *Mov Disord*. 2014;29:437–43.

Lu CS, Thompson PD, Quinn NP, Parkes JD, Marsden CD. Ramsay Hunt syndrome and coeliac disease: a new association? *Mov Disord*. 1986;1:209–19.

Video 55.1

Stimulus-sensitive myoclonus is shown both in upper and lower limbs. There is also action myoclonus when the patient attempts to put his socks on and gait ataxia without limb ataxia.

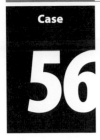

Asymmetric Myoclonus and Apraxia: Corticobasal Syndrome

Roberto Erro, Maria Stamelou, and Kailash P. Bhatia

Clinical History

This 69-year-old right-handed woman with no family history was admitted to our department because of a 3-year history of involuntary jerks of her left arm and leg when touching something or on action. She further reported that her left hand dexterity had deteriorated over the past few months, so that she had difficulties using her left hand to comb her hair or for make-up. There were no other major complaints; in particular, her memory and sleep were normal. However, she was feeling low in mood.

Examination

On examination, eye movements and cranial nerves were found to be normal. There were stimulus-sensitive jerks of her left arm and leg when outstretched (see Video 56.1). Moreover, there was mild bradykinesia on finger tapping with the left hand and she had difficulties coping gestures with the same hand. The remaining neurological examination was normal.

General Remarks

Although structural lesions should be always excluded when symptoms are confined to one side of the body, the combination of cortical (i.e. myoclonus and apraxia) and sub-cortical (i.e. bradykinesia) signs with an asymmetric (or unilateral) distribution in a patient of this age is very suggestive of CBS.

Investigations and Diagnosis

Standard biochemical investigations and a brain MRI were within normal limits. A standard EEG was proven to be normal, while an electrophysiological study of her jerks showed their duration to be between 25 and 50 ms, associated with episodes of sudden loss of muscle tone lasting up to 100 ms. There was a definite pyramidal pattern of activation at adequate latency, and a jerk-locked EEG back-averaging showed a pre-movement potential about 20 ms before the jerks of the left first dorsal interossei muscle. SSEPs from the left limbs were enlarged (N20-P25 amplitude of 34.2 microvolts). Altogether, the electrophysiological features were consistent with a cortical origin of the myoclonus. A DaT-Scan was proven to be abnormal, with reduced uptake in the right striatum. She was therefore diagnosed with CBS.

Special Remarks

CBS is the term which is used clinically in cases like the current one since the underlying pathology can be that of CBD as well as of PSP, AD, and other neurodegenerative diseases. Although the classical description of CBS (as associated to CDB, cf. Case 8) encompasses a very asymmetric parkinsonian syndrome, with marked bradykinesia and dystonia, it can also present with myoclonus and minimal extrapyramidal symptoms. In fact, it has been shown that myoclonus is indeed more common than dystonia in pathologically proven CBD cases. The myoclonus observed in CBS is classically focal, confined to one limb (usually the arm) and is most prominent on voluntary action or in response to sensory stimulation. Examination reveals that the myoclonus can occur at rest but EMG recordings reveals that apparently spontaneous myoclonus often occurs on a background of continuous muscle activity due to the presence of rigidity and dystonia. Although in some cases (as in this patient), electrophysiological characteristics of myoclonus support a cortical origin, a slightly different underlying pathophysiology with enhancement of a direct sensory input to the motor cortex is speculated to be the main mechanism. As stated, this phenotype is highly suggestive of CBS. However, there is a rare entity of late onset asymmetric idiopathic myoclonus, which may come into the differential diagnosis of cases who have cortical myoclonus with onset later than 65 years of age, without dementia and other clinical features suggestive of a progressive neurodegenerative disorder or other secondary causes of myoclonus. In this syndrome (e.g. late onset asymmetric idiopathic myoclonus) there are neither clinical nor imaging evidence of basal ganglia dysfunction, but what this entity represents remains not clearly defined.

Suggested Readings

Katschnig P, Massano J, Edwards MJ, Schwingenschuh P, Cordivari C, Bhatia KP. Late-onset asymmetric myoclonus: an emerging syndrome. *Mov Disord.* 2011;26:1744–8.

Stamelou M, Alonso-Canovas A, Bhatia KP. Dystonia in corticobasal degeneration: a review of the literature on 404 pathologically proven cases. *Mov Disord.* 2012;27:696–702.

Thompson PD, Day BL, Rothwell JC, Brown P, Britton TC, Marsden CD. The myoclonus in corticobasal degeneration. Evidence for two forms of cortical reflex myoclonus. *Brain.* 1994;117:1197–207.

  Video 56.1

The video shows bradykinesia on finger tapping with the right hand. Stimulus-sensitive myoclonus of the right limbs as well as apraxia of the right hand are shown.

Rapidly Progressive Cognitive Regression and Myoclonus: New Variant CJD

Roberto Erro and Kailash P. Bhatia

Clinical History

This 36-year-old British woman, who had been generally in good health, was admitted in our hospital for an 8-month history of progressive involuntary jerks, balance difficulties, and severe cognitive deterioration and behaviour regression, so that her memory and language were dramatically impaired and she started doing unusual things, including bringing a teddy bear with her all the time, and adopted childish mannerisms. Also, she had emotional lability and severe anxiety.

Examination

She was alert but not fully collaborative, so that examination was very limited. There were spontaneous myoclonic jerks in her upper limbs on posture. Moreover, she had oral, trunk, and upper limbs stereotypes and mannerism. She was not orientated and was inappropriate in her answers.

General Remarks

Although this patient presented with movement disorders including myoclonus and mannerism/stereotypies, her clinical phenotype was dominated by a marked cognitive impairment and behavioural symptoms. The differential diagnosis of rapidly developing cognitive impairment with psychiatric features includes prion disease, immune-mediate disorders including NMDA-receptor encephalitis or paraneoplastic encephalitis, toxic or metabolic causes and infective disease, including HIV-related encephalopathy and Whipple's disease. The diagnostic work-up should be accordingly very broad.

Investigations and Diagnosis

Extensive biochemical investigations, including tests for autoimmune disorders and EEG, showed generalized slow wave activity, with no pseudo-periodic pattern. A brain MRI showed generalized atrophy (see Figure 57.1A). Moreover, on FLAIR sequences demonstrated bilateral increased signal in the posterior thalamus (i.e. the pulvinar sign, see Figure 57.1B). CSF 14-3-3 protein was raised and she was found to have the MM genotype at codon 129 of the *PRNP* gene. A tonsillar biopsy demonstrated the presence of PrP^{Sc}, thus confirming the diagnosis of new variant CJD (vCJD).

Special Remarks

vCJD was first described as a distinct neuropathological entity associated with BSE, commonly known as mad cow disease, in 1996. The early features of vCDJ are non-specific, often with psychiatric and behavioural changes, including depression, anxiety, social withdrawal, emotional lability, aggression, insomnia, and hallucinations, and in some cases with sensory changes. Prominent early features in some patients are in fact dysaesthesiae or pain in the limb or face. The progression is dramatic and all cases develop within few months marked with cognitive impairment with akinetic mutism. Movement disorders, and specifically myoclonus, are seen in most patients, and chorea is also often present, along with cerebellar ataxia. Ocular abnormalities and cortical blindness also have been reported. vCDJ has a relatively longer prognosis compared to other prion diseases, median disease duration being of 14 months.

The EEG is always abnormal, but does not show the typical pseudo-periodic pattern observed in sporadic CJD. The hyperintensity of the pulvinar on T2 sequences called the 'pulvinar sign' is seen in the majority of cases, usually as a late feature. However, it is not specific for vCJD, as it can be seen also in both sporadic CJD and limbic encephalitis, both of which should be considered in the differential diagnosis. Tonsillar biopsy is a sensitive and specific procedure for the diagnosis of vCJD, since PrP^{Sc} is uniformly present in clinically affected patients but not in other human forms of prion disease. A positive tonsillar biopsy obviates the need for brain biopsy. *PRNP* mutation analyses

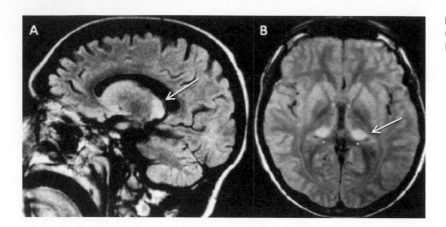

Figure 57.1 T1-weighted sagittal (A) and axial (B) sequences showing the pulvinar sign (arrows).

should be performed in all cases suspected to have vCJD to exclude the inherited forms of prion disease.

Suggested Readings

Corato M, Cereda C, Cova E, Ferrarese C, Ceroni M. Young-onset CJD: age and disease phenotype in variant and sporadic forms. *Funct Neurol.* 2006;21:211–15.

Day GS, Tang-Wai DF. When dementia progresses quickly: a practical approach to the diagnosis and management of rapidly progressive dementia. *Neurodegener Dis Manag.* 2014;4:41–56.

Takada LT, Geschwind MD. Prion diseases. *Semin Neurol.* 2013;33:348–56.

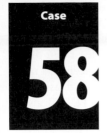

Familial Cortical 'Tremor'

Roberto Erro and Kailash P. Bhatia

Clinical History

This 35-year old right-handed man had been diagnosed with epilepsy by the age of 7–8 years, having had a few GTCS. He has been on carbamazepine with good results since then. Over the years, he tried to spontaneously stop carbamazepine and this brought on a few seizures. He has been hence started again on anti-epileptic drugs and has been fine for the subsequent years. By the age of 21 years, he noted a twitching on the right side of his face. At the same time, he also developed a stutter. Around the age of 29, his twitching spread into his right arm, especially on action (for instance, upon writing). For this reason, he sought medical advice and was tried on different anti-epileptics, which were not helpful, despite his epilepsy being still well controlled.

As to his family history, his parents were fine, but his sister (aged 41) was diagnosed with ET as well as his half-sister (aged 23), who also had epilepsy.

Examination

On examination (see Video 58.1), eye movements and cranial nerves were found to be normal. He had myoclonic twitches on the right side of the face, mainly in the lower part, when speaking. His voice was affected in the way that he tended to stutter when he was having his facial twitches, but no stuttering was present otherwise. He had a fine jerky tremor of his both arms on posture and of his right one when writing. A fine tremor could be appreciated in his lower limbs. Myoclonic jerks were evident in his lower limbs when he was asked to stand on one leg. The remaining neurological examination was normal.

General Remarks

The combination of myoclonic jerks (mimicking a tremor in the limbs) with epilepsy, the positive family history, the benign phenotype with relatively slow or absent progression, and the absence of other features, including cognitive impairment, is very suggestive of FCMTE. In our case, the localization of the myoclonic twitches in his face was of great value in interpreting his limb tremor as myoclonic and raises the suspicion that the diagnosis of ET in his sisters was wrong. Electrophysiological testing of the jerks can be of great value in this regard and also to differential between cortical and sub-cortical myoclonus, allowing the differential diagnosis with DYT11 (cf. Case 53). Patients may easily be misdiagnosed as having JME due to the co-existence of myoclonic jerks and GTCS. However, JME differs clinically from FCMTE because of the absence of cortical tremor, the mainly proximal myoclonic jerks, and seizures typically occurring at awakening. On the other hand side, the benign phenotype and progression, with the absence of other system involvement, clearly differentiate FCMTE from other myoclonic disorders, including PME (cf. Cases 53 and 54) and only rarely an extensive diagnostic work-up is required.

Investigations and Diagnosis

Standard blood investigations and a brain MRI were normal. A routine EEG was also found to be normal. P25-N35 amplitude of cortical somatosensory-evoked potentials was enlarged (Figure 58.1A), supporting the presence of giant-evoked potentials. Moreover, the C-reflex was present (Figure 58.1B). Multichannel EEG/EMG recording showed continuous rhythmic jerks with a frequency up to 20 Hz when holding the right upper limb against gravity or during action, along with brief episodes of loss of tone. The jerk duration was about 20 ms and there was a typical pyramidal progression of the jerks. Altogether, these features were consistent with cortical myoclonus. The patient was therefore diagnosed with FCMTE and switched on levetiracetam (1,500 mg day) with a good response on his myoclonic jerks.

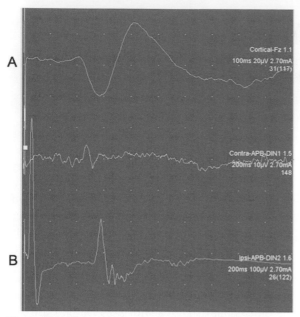

Figure 58.1 (A) Giant SSEPs over the left hemisphere; (B) presence of the C-reflex, elicited after the stimulation of the median nerve. A black and white version of this figure will appear in some formats. For the colour version, please refer to the plate section.

Special Remarks

FCMTE is a variably inherited syndrome character-ized by cortical limb tremors, myoclonic jerks, and occasional generalized or focal seizures with a non-progressive or very slowly progressive disease course, and no signs of early dementia or cerebellar ataxia.

Onset of FCMTE is usually in the second decade of life (but age of onset can range from age 11 to 50) with a minor cortical hand tremor. The myoclonic tremor consists of continuous, arrhythmic fine twitching in the hands that is exacerbated by fatigue or emotional stress. Often, there is no progression of severity in these tremors until late adulthood. Myoclonus can also manifest as arrhythmic, segmental jerks of the upper limbs heightened by posture and action. Rare tonic-clonic seizures are also a manifestation of FCMTE, often occurring after the appearance of tremors and myoclonus and precipitated by photic stimulation, emotional stress, and sleep deprivation.

Two genes – *CNTN2* (encoding contactin 2, muta-tions of which are transmitted in a recessive fashion) and *ACMSD* (encoding a critical enzyme of the kynure-nine pathway of the tryptophan metabolism, muta-tions of which are transmitted dominantly) – have

been reported in single families and wait for further confirmation. The genetic heterogeneity of FCMTE (which is usually transmitted dominantly with a sup-posed high penetrance) is high and at least four differ-ent genetic loci have been identified. Recently, a novel mutation in *PLA2G6* has been identified as causa-tive in a Chinese pedigree with FCMTE and awaits confirmation

Unlike ET, it has a poor response to beta-blockers but improves with antiepileptic drugs. Alcohol aggravates this tremor and hence should be avoided. Valproate, levetiracetam, and benzodiazepines are most beneficial in the treatment of cortical tremors and myoclonus due to their combined antiepileptic and antimyoclonic effects. In very rare instances, epilepsy may be difficult to treat.

Suggested Readings

Cen Z, Huang C, Yin H, et al. Clinical and neurophysiological features of familial cortical myoclonic tremor with epilepsy. *Mov Disord*. 2016;31:1704–1710.

Gao L, Li L, Ye J, et al. Identification of a novel mutation in PLA2G6 gene in a Chinese pedigree with familial cortical myoclonic tremor with epilepsy. *Seizure*. 2016;41:81–5.

Martí-Massó JF, Bergareche A, Makarov V, et al. The ACMSD gene, involved in tryptophan metabolism, is mutated in a family with cortical myoclonus, epilepsy, and parkinsonism. *J Mol Med (Berl)*. 2013;91:1399–406.

Stogmann E, Reinthaler E, Eltawil S, et al. Autosomal recessive cortical myoclonic tremor and epilepsy: association with a mutation in the potassium channel associated gene CNTN2. *Brain*. 2013;136:1155–60.

van Rootselaar AF, van Schaik IN, van den Maagdenberg AM, et al. Familial cortical myoclonic tremor with epilepsy: a single syndromic classification for a group of pedigrees bearing common features. *Mov Disord*. 2005;20:665–73.

   Video 58.1

This patient has myoclonic twitches on the right side of the face, mainly in the lower part, when speaking. His voice is also affected in the way that he tends to stutter when his facial twitches occur. He has a fine jerky tremor of his both arms on posture. Myoclonic jerks are evident in his lower limbs when he is asked to stand on one leg.

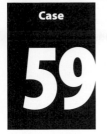

Case

59

Prominent Myoclonus and Parkinsonism in MSA

Roberto Erro, Maria Stamelou, and Kailash P. Bhatia

Clinical History

This 72-year-old right-handed retired civil engineer was referred to us with a working diagnosis of parkinsonism. His initial symptoms were tremor in the right hand, which made it difficult to place the golf ball on the tee 3 years earlier. He then noticed 'weakness' in his legs, more on the right, and within 12 months the right extremity tremor was interfering with other daily activities, including shaving, writing, and eating. He reported that his tremor was worse with action and much less at rest. He further noticed a decline in dexterity in the right hand for doing up buttons and cufflinks, and deterioration in his speech. Moreover, he has had symptoms of urinary hesitancy, dribbling, and urinary urgency with frequent nocturia for at least 3 years. His 'shakiness' progressively worsened and spread to his legs, so that his walking was impaired and he had to use a wheelchair. No other symptoms were reported.

He had been for a year or so on levodopa treatment (300 mg daily) without any clear improvement of his symptoms.

Examination

On examination, it was found that he was hypomimic and his speech was slurred. There was no classic pill-rolling tremor as such, but a myoclonic tremor could be observed on posture (Video 59.1). This was evident also in his legs when they were hold against gravity. His tongue was also trembling when protruded outside his mouth. Moreover, he had bilateral bradykinesia in both upper and lower limbs. He had some leg jerks on standing, thus producing some unsteadiness, but postural reflexes were normal as such. His gait was short-stepped and wide based. Lower limb reflexes were brisk. The remaining neurological examination was unremarkable.

General Remarks

The presence of a parkinsonian syndrome, apparently unresponsive to levodopa, along with mild cerebellar signs and with the further development of possible autonomic dysfunction is suggestive of MSA (cf. Cases 8 and 62). At disease onset, the differentiation between a classic pill-rolling tremor and myoclonus would have been useful in the differential diagnosis. Myoclonus is in fact very unusual in PD (and usually associated with medications including amantadine) and would rather favour a diagnosis of an atypical parkinsonism. In this regard, an autonomic evaluation and a detailed brain MRI would prove useful to make the correct diagnosis.

Investigations and Diagnosis

A brain MRI showed cerebellar and pons atrophy, while a DaT-Scan was proven to be abnormal. A cardiovascular autonomic function assessment (cardiac response to deep breathing, cardiovascular response to the Valsalva manoeuvre, and cardiovascular response to upright tilt) revealed the presence of moderate autonomic dysfunction. He was therefore eventually diagnosed with probable MSA, according to current clinical criteria.

Special Remarks

The 'tremor' observed in MSA patients is often atypical and takes the form of an irregular, jerky, postural tremor of the arms. Also, discrete myoclonic jerks of the fingers and/or toes, sometimes stimulus-sensitive, can be present both at rest and on action, usually in more advanced stages of the disease. Myoclonus has been described to occur in up to 31 per cent of MSA patients and it is seen as small-amplitude, non-rhythmic movements involving distal fingers (i.e. poly-minimyoclonus) or more rarely the whole hand or arm (as in our case), occurring on posture or on action but not at rest, is typical of MSA rather than of PD. In fact, accelerometric recordings show small-amplitude oscillations that, in contrast to what is seen in patients with true tremor, do not have predominant peak in the Fast Fourier frequency spectrum analysis. Moreover, these jerks have the electrophysiological characteristics of cortical reflex myoclonus.

Suggested Readings

Okuma Y, Fujishima K, Miwa H, Mori H, Mizuno Y. Myoclonic tremulous movements in multiple system atrophy are a form of cortical myoclonus. *Mov Disord.* 2005;20:451–6.

Salazar G, Valls-Solé J, Martí MJ, Chang H, Tolosa ES. Postural and action myoclonus in patients with parkinsonian type multiple system atrophy. *Mov Disord.* 2000;15:77–83.

Wenning GK, Ben Shlomo Y, Magalhães M, Daniel SE, Quinn NP. Clinical features and natural history of multiple system atrophy. An analysis of 100 cases. *Brain.* 1994;117:835–45.

Video 59.1

There is a myoclonic tremor on posture of his arms and legs. Furthermore, his tongue shakes when protruded.

Case

60

Functional Axial Myoclonus

Roberto Erro and Carla Cordivari

Clinical History

This 63-year-old, right-handed, man with no family history for any neurological disorders was referred to our department for an 18-month history of jerks involving mainly his trunk and to a lesser extent his legs, which occurred at rest without any triggers. His jerks were present when sitting or lying down but not when standing, and were interfering significantly with his daily activities and affecting his sleep. His symptoms could fluctuate in severity, but he reported a significant worsening over time.

Examination

On examination (see Video 60.1), the only abnormal finding was that of abnormal jerks of his trunk that could at times spread to his lower limbs. His jerks were stereotyped and consisted of flexor axial spams of brief duration, which could occur also in cluster. The remaining neurological examination was entirely normal.

General Remarks

Axial 'myoclonic' jerks can be classified into two broad groups: SSM or PSM, according to the putative spinal circuitry involved. Both are generally resistant to supraspinal influences such as sleep (and hence can persist in sleep) or voluntary action (and hence can be present at rest). SSM is usually symptomatic of an underlying structural lesion such as syringomyelia, myelitis, spinal cord trauma, vascular lesion, or malignancy, and is by definition confined to one or a few contiguous myotomes, and therefore is unlikely in this patient, in whom the jerks affected many myotomes from the upper trunk to the lower limbs. The clinical picture would fit in with a diagnosis of PSM. PSM has been described to be a form of spinal myoclonus where a spinal generator recruits axial muscles up and down the spinal cord via long and slow propriospinal pathways. However, there have been recently some issues regarding the clinical diagnosis of PSM on the basis of

electrophysiological tests, which are therefore required to establish the diagnosis.

Investigations and Diagnosis

A whole spine was normal. A multichannel EMG–EEG recording showed a constant pattern of muscle activation with the upper rectus abdominis muscle always firing first, and a slow conduction velocity of about 7 m/s, determined from the inter-bursts interval of the myoclonic activity, which would be consistent with a diagnosis of PSM. However, jerk-locked back averaging of the EEG traces showed the presence of a Bereitschaftspotential (BP; from German, 'readiness potential', also called the premotor potential; Figure 60.1) preceding the jerks and supporting strong electrophysiological evidence of a psychogenic nature for the jerks.

Special Remarks

It has been increasingly recognized that a number of patients with a diagnosis of idiopathic PSM have either a subsequent clinical course or electrophysiological features indicating that the likely etiology is psychogenic. There is in fact considerable uncertainty about the possibility of reaching a firm diagnosis of idiopathic PSM on a clinical basis alone and in this regard electrophysiology is mandatory. Polymyographic recording matched with EEG can in fact show either an incongruent EMG pattern for PSM or reveal the presence of a BP. If, on the one hand, the presence of a BP strongly supports the diagnosis of a psychogenic movement disorder, on the other hand, its absence does not exclude this possibility, since the absence of BP may reflect technical difficulties inherent in the test, and the BP can be affected by the level of intention, motivation, and attention as well as the complexity of the movement.

An attempt to describe the clinical features of psychogenic axial jerks showed that there could be a

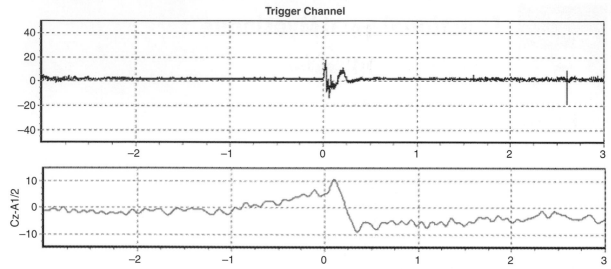

Figure 60.1 Jerk-locked EEG back averaging showing a negative shift with amplitude of more than 5 microvolts over the central cortical areas, starting about 1 second before the jerks (i.e. the bereitschaftspotential). A black and white version of this figure will appear in some formats. For the colour version, please refer to the plate section.

number of clinical clues suggesting a psychogenic etiology, even when electrophysiology cannot be performed. These include predominant involvement of the lower limbs, facial involvement, and unilateral involvement of the limbs. Yet, clinical classification of axial jerks can be very difficult in single patients and hence, if electrophysiology is not available, prolonged observation and long-term follow-up might prove useful to distinguishing organic from psychogenic axial jerks.

Suggested Readings

Erro R, Bhatia KP, Edwards MJ, Farmer SF, Cordivari C. Clinical diagnosis of propriospinal myoclonus is unreliable: an electrophysiologic study. *Mov Disord.* 2013;28:1868–73.

Erro R, Edwards MJ, Bhatia KP, et al. Psychogenic axial myoclonus: clinical features and long-term outcome. *Parkinsonism Relat Disord.* 2014;20:596–9.

van der Salm SM, Erro R, Cordivari C, et al. Propriospinal myoclonus: clinical reappraisal and review of literature. *Neurology.* 2014;83:1862–70.

 Video 60.1

This patient has repetitive jerks originating from the trunk and propagating to his lower limbs.

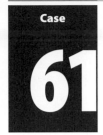

Slowly Progressive Unsteadiness and Double Vision: SCA6

Roberto Erro and Kailash P. Bhatia

Clinical History

A 57-year-old woman with no family history was referred for a long-standing unsteadiness. She mentioned that in her late thirties she started feeling unsteady and veering off to one side inconsistently. However, her symptoms were minor and very slowly progressive so that she did not seek medical advice. Recently, she occasionally started having double vision and when reading, she would see 'the words jumping'. Moreover, she found herself to be clumsy with her upper limbs as well.

Examination

On examination, it was found that she had spontaneous down-beat nystagmus as well as gaze-evoked nystagmus. Smooth pursuit was broken. There was a possible telangiectasia in her bulbar conjunctiva. There was no dysarthria. There was no appendicular ataxia, but she had mild dysdiadochokinesia. Her gait was mildly broad-based and unsteady and she had extreme difficulties in tandem-walking. The remaining neurological examination was normal.

General Remarks

The complaint of our patient seeing 'words jumping' when reading is consistent with oscillopsia, which is defined as an illusion of an unstable vision, made up of the perception of to-and-fro movement of the environment. There are a number of peripheral and central disorders that can result in oscillopsia. In our patients, however, there was a clear spontaneous and positional nystagmus on examination, accounting for her oscillopsia. The combination of nystagmus with gait ataxia is indicative of a cerebellar disorder. On examination, a telangiectasia in her bulbar conjunctiva was seen, thus raising the suspicion of ATM. However, the age at onset and the long disease course with a benign progression was against this diagnosis (cf. Case 65). Obviously, a number of acquired conditions should be considered,

including alcohol or drug-related ataxia, vitamin deficiency, coeliac disease, vascular disease, primary or metastatic tumors, and paraneoplastic cerebellar syndromes. On the contrary, even in the absence of a family history, the most common types of SCA (particularly those presenting with a 'pure' cerebellar phenotype without involvement of other systems) should be considered in the differential diagnosis.

Investigations and Diagnosis

An extensive set of biochemical investigation to exclude secondary causes of ataxia was normal while a brain MRI showed clear cerebellar atrophy. Genetic testing for the most common forms of SCA were pursued and she was found to carry a CAG-repeat expansion in the *CACNA1A* gene, thus confirming the diagnosis of SCA6.

Special Remarks

SCA6 is characterized by adult onset, slowly progressive cerebellar ataxia, dysarthria, and nystagmus, with onset usually ranging from 43 to 52 years. Yet, age of onset and clinical picture vary even within the same family and sibs with the same size full-penetrance allele may differ in the age of onset by as many as 12 years. The most common symptoms at presentation are gait unsteadiness and imbalance, while only a minority of patients complain about dysarthria. Visual disturbances may also occur and result from diplopia, difficulty fixating on moving objects, horizontal gaze-evoked nystagmus, and vertical nystagmus. The disorder is slowly progressive, but eventually all affected subjects have gait ataxia, upper-limb incoordination, intention tremor, and dysarthria, and at the very last stage, dysphagia can also occur. SCA6 is considered one of the purest types of SCA. However, hyperreflexia and extensor plantar responses are seen in up to half of the affected patients, while dystonia occurs in about 25 per cent. Because the phenotypic manifestations are not specific, the diagnosis of SCA6 rests on molecular genetic testing, showing an expanded polymorphic CAG repeat in exon 47 of the *CACNA1A* gene (normal: 18 or fewer repeats). Very interestingly, missense mutations of *CACNA1A* are responsible for different disorders, including EA type 2 and FHM. Despite their well-described phenotypes, SCA6, EA2, and FHM demonstrate some clinical overlap and it is not uncommon that SCA6 patients complain about an episodic (or fluctuating) course at onset.

Suggested Readings

Rossi M, Perez-Lloret S, Cerquetti D, et al. Movement disorders in autosomal dominant cerebellar aaxias: a systematic review. *Mov Disord Clin Pract.* 2014;1:154–60.

Solodkin A, Gomez CM. Spinocerebellar ataxia type 6. *Handb Clin Neurol.* 2012;103:461–73.

Case

62

Cerebellar Ataxia with Urinary Incontinence: MSA-C

Roberto Erro and Kailash P. Bhatia

Clinical History

A 60-year-old woman with no family history was referred for a 3-year history of difficulties using her right hand and unsteadiness. At onset, she had difficulty using her right hand, which was clumsy. This slowly worsened and after a year she developed episodes of dizziness and progressive balance problems leading her to use a wheelchair. She also developed speech and swallowing difficulty as well as urinary urgency and occasional incontinence. The episodes of dizziness occurred mainly when she stood up from sitting.

Examination

On examination (see Video 62.1), it was found that she had broken smooth pursuit, hypopetric saccades, and a scanning speech. There was bradykinesia both on finger and foot tapping (more severe on the right than on the left). There were cerebellar features of bilateral upper limb ataxia with dysdiadochokinesis bilaterally. There were some finger jerks. Gait was short stepped, but also wide based. The remaining neurological examination was normal, apart from brisk reflexes in her lower limbs.

Investigations and Diagnosis

A brain MRI showed a marked cerebellar and pons atrophy (Figure 62.1), with the 'hot cross bun sign' (cf. Figure 8.1B). A DaT-Scan was performed which showed bilateral tracer binding reduction in the putamen nucleus. An autonomic evaluation confirmed evidence of cardiovascular autonomic failure (resting blood pressure was 168/62 which fell within one minute of tilt to 60/41). Thus, a diagnosis of MSA-C was made.

Remarks

The combination of cerebellar features with dysautonomia and parkinsonism is highly suggestive of MSA-C

and the diagnostic work-up should be performed accordingly. Indeed, in our case, a positive DaT-Scan along with the presence of cerebellar and parkinsonian signs as well as dysautonomia led to the diagnosis of MSA-C. Furthermore, her brain MRI showing atrophy of the pons and cerebellum and the presence of the 'hot-cross bun' sign was also in keeping with MSA. The cerebellar variant of MSA is less common than its parkinsonian counterpart, at least in Europe and North America. In the Far-East population such a trend seems to be inverted, probably reflecting a different genetic or environmental background. Whether the phenotypes of MSA-P and MSA-C differentially affect survival is controversial, but it has been suggested that MSA-C is somewhat more benign and has a longer survival. Yet, often patients show a mixed phenotype with both parkinsonism and a cerebellar syndrome, as in our case.

While a general overview of MSA has been provided in Case 8, we will here focus on the differential diagnosis of MSA-C. In fact, some types of SCAs, particularly SCA2 and SCA3 (also known as Machado–Joseph disease), can present with a cerebellar syndrome with additional autonomic dysfunction and, possibly, mild parkinsonism. MRI can also show the "hot-cross bun" sign, which is not specific to MSA. FXTAS syndrome should be also considered (cf. Case 63), even if very rare in women. The mechanism thereby FXTAS develops in women is due to skewed X-inactivation, with a greater fraction of cells expressing an active permutation. Additional clues pointing towards the FXTAS diagnosis are neuropathy and infertility or premature menopause.

Another condition to include in the differential diagnosis is CANVAS syndrome, which can very often encompass automonic failure and hence mimic the cerebellar variant of MSA. The pathognomonic feature of this condition is an impaired vestibulo-ocular reflex. Finally, for a number of patients, a conclusive diagnosis cannot be reached and they are usually grouped into the rubric of ILOCA, but the newly available genetic

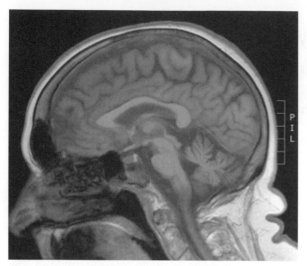

Figure 62.1 Sagittal MRI T1-weighted sequence showing volume loss in the pons and cerebellum.

approaches will likely allow the reclassification of a number of these cases into specific disease entities.

Suggested Readings

Lin DJ, Hermann KL, Schmahmann JD. Multiple system atrophy of the cerebellar type: clinical state of the art. *Mov Disord*. 2014;29:294–304.

Wenning GK, Kraft E, Beck RW, et al. Cerebellar presentation of multiple system atrophy. *Mov Disord*. 1997;12:115–17.

Video 62.1

She has a scanning speech and broken smooth pursuit. There is bradykinesia on finger tapping bilaterally. Limb ataxia is shown on finger–nose test. Her gait is short stepped, but also wide based.

63

Progressive Ataxia, Tremor, Autonomic Dysfunction, and Cognitive Impairment: FXTAS

Roberto Erro, Maria Stamelou, and Kailash P. Bhatia

Clinical History

This 69-year-old man has a long history, spanning over 15 years, of bilateral tremor of his hands, present both at rest and on action, and poor balance with associated falls. Besides these complaints, his wife reported that he could get lost while driving and that he could occasionally forget names of distant family members. During the past 5 years, he has further suffered from 'dizzy episodes', which usually occurred on standing. Moreover, he has urinary urgency with occasional incontinence and does not have spontaneous erections.

Examination

On examination (Video 63.1), it was found that ocular pursuits were broken and the saccadic eye movements were slow. Inspection of the upper limbs revealed a tremor at rest with mild asymmetry, being more prominent on the right than the left. On assessment of posture, some jerky elements to the tremor were found. On intention and action, the tremor was more prominent on the right, and during the index-nose test, a mild dysmetria could be seen. Moreover, there was mild rigidity and slowing on repetitive movements, which was more prominent in the right upper limb than the left. His gait was slightly wide based and short stepped. A bedside MMSE was performed which yielded a score of 16/30. Finally, pinprick and vibration sensations were reduced to the ankles bilaterally, whereas the remaining neurological examination was normal.

General Remarks

The syndromic association of parkinsonism with cerebellar signs and autonomic dysfunction could raise the suspicion of MSA-C (cf. Case 62). However, there are some red-flags in this case which would not entirely fit with the latter. First, disease duration of more than 15 years is against a diagnosis of MSA, where one would expect a severer progression with more prominent autonomic signs. Second, the evidence of

memory issues is also unusual for MSA, where a certain degree of cognitive impairment can be seen, but has usually a frontal/sub-cortical pattern. Finally, the presence of a possible neuropathy is also helpful in the differential diagnosis and in fact, among the disorders to be considered, this particular association of cerebellar and parkinsonian signs, autonomic and cognitive dysfunction, along with neuropathy should raise the suspicion of FXTAS.

Investigations and Diagnosis

Brain MRI revealed generalized volume loss and mild cerebellar atrophy. Moreover, T2 hyperintensities involving the middle cerebellar peduncles bilaterally were observed (Figure 63.1). A DaT-Scan was performed and it was abnormal. Genetic screening for the *FMR1* gene was performed and he was found to have 90 CGG repeats (normal: <55; pre-mutation: 55–200; mutation: >200), leading to the diagnosis of FXTAS.

Special Remarks

FXTAS is a late onset (onset usually occurs after age 50 years) neurodegenerative disorder, occurring in carriers of a premutation CGG repeat expansion in the *FMR1* gene. The penetrance of FXTAS in male carriers over 50 years old is about 40 per cent, while only 20 per cent of female carriers develop neurological signs. The typical FXTAS phenotype usually features the combination of intention tremor and ataxia. However, tremor is not always present and some patients with *FMR1* pre-mutations may appear by history and examination to have a pure rigid-akinetic syndrome. In most cases, however, additional signs are present and the main differential diagnosis is with MSA-C and SCAs. A family history of mental retardation or premature ovarian failure provides important clues. However, it has been recently shown that up to 43 per cent of the FXTAS patients have no family history of FXTAS syndrome. In terms of syndromic association, the presence of early

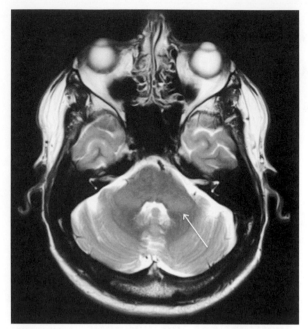

Figure 63.1 Axial MRI T2-weighted sequence showing the 'MCP sign' bilaterally (hyperintensity of the middle cerebellar peduncles, white arrow).

callosum splenium hyperintensity can also be seen and, according to one study, it is as frequent (68 per cent) as the MCP sign (64 per cent). Dopaminergic functional imaging can be normal in FXTAS. Thus, an MSA phenotype with normal dopaminergic imaging should raise suspicion for FXTAS, but an abnormal scan does not exclude this rare diagnosis.

Suggested Readings

Apartis E, Blancher A, Meissner WG, et al. FXTAS: new insights and the need for revised diagnostic criteria. *Neurology*. 2012;79:1898–907.

Kamm C, Healy DG, Quinn NP, et al. The fragile X tremor ataxia syndrome in the differential diagnosis of multiple system atrophy: data from the EMSA Study Group. *Brain*. 2005;128(Pt 8):1855–60.

Renaud M, Perriard J, Coudray S, et al. Relevance of corpus callosum splenium versus middle cerebellar peduncle hyperintensity for FXTAS diagnosis in clinical practice. *J Neurol*. 2015;262:435–42.

  Video 63.1

A bilateral, though asymmetric, irregular tremor is seen at rest, on posture, and action. Moreover, there is general hypokinesia, although it is difficult to judge whether there is decrement on finger tapping, also because tremor frequency tends to take over during finger tapping. Gait is unstable and reflects a combination of parkinsonian and ataxic features.

cognitive dysfunction and clinically detectable peripheral neuropathy (that are not usually present in MSA) are probably the most useful clues. Investigation-wise, MRI findings in FXTAS are those of increased signal intensity in the middle cerebellar peduncles on T2-weighted images or FLAIR sequences (the so-called MCP sign, which is seen in nearly 60 per cent of the cases). Corpus

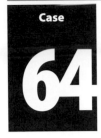

Case

64

Sensory Ataxic Neuropathy with Dysarthria and Ophthalmoparesis (SANDO) Syndrome

Roberto Erro, Amit Batla, and Kailash P. Bhatia

Clinical History

A 64-year-old male patient, with no past or family history of relevance, initially sought medical care at the age of 30 years, because of the presence of tingling and numbness in his lower limbs. A nerve conduction study revealed a large fibre sensory neuropathy. His symptoms worsened over time, affecting his gait, but he could walk unaided and carried on his employment. Aged 40, he further developed slurring of speech and, when assessed at the age of 55, eye movement abnormalities consistent with external ophthalmoplegia were noted. Aged 57, he additionally developed a rest tremor on his right hand and in the following 3 years, his mobility worsened to such an extent that he was significantly confined and could only walk for short distances with the support of a frame. Owing to the presence of these new symptoms, he was referred to our department.

Examination

Ocular movements were markedly restricted with absent Bell's phenomenon, consistent with external ophthalmoplegia (see Video 64.1). He had facial hypomimia, and his speech was dysarthric. There was a rest tremor of the right hand with re-emergence on posture, along with bradykinesia on both finger- and foot-tapping tasks (right>left) and rigidity. His walking (with support) was slow and ataxic, but he further had freezing of gait on turning. Postural reflexes were clearly impaired. In addition, reflexes were all absent, but the right biceps jerk. He had reduced pinprick sensation distally in his lower limbs up to the knees bilaterally. Vibration sense was also reduced up to the costal margin on the right and iliac crest on the left.

General Remarks

Although the clinical picture in this case is quite complex with a constellation of symptoms and signs, the clinical distinction between sensory and cerebellar ataxia (and the further absence of other cerebellar signs) allowed us to exclude cerebellar disorders, including some types of SCA, which can also present with ataxia, neuropathy, dysarthria, oculomotor disturbances, and parkinsonism. Instead, the oculomotor findings (chronic external ophthalmoplegia) are critical here and narrow the differential diagnosis to mitochondrial disorders. Moreover, the presence of Sensory Ataxic Neuropathy and Dysarthria, along with Ophthalmoplegia, amounts to what has been referred to as SANDO syndrome, which can be due to mutations of either nuclear mithocondrial genes or mitochondrial DNA (mtDNA). On the basis of the oculomotor findings, the main differential diagnosis would have been with neuromuscular junction disorders. In the latter, however, one would not have expected the presence of additional sensory ataxia and parkinsonism.

Investigations and Diagnosis

Neurophysiological testing confirmed an axonal polyneuropathy. His brain MRI was normal, whereas a DaT-Scan was abnormal. On the basis of SANDO phenotype and the presence of parkinsonism (SANDO-P), he was tested for common *POLG* gene mutations. He was found to be compound heterozygous for c.1399G>A (p.Ala467Thr) and c.2243G>C (p.Trp748Ser), the autosomal recessive pathogenic variants of *POLG*.

Special Remarks

SANDO syndrome is one of the clinical presentations of chronic PEO, a mitochondrial disorder, which by definition is characterized by slowly progressive paralysis of the extraocular muscles, whereas ciliary and iris muscles are not involved. SANDO syndrome is a rare disorder with less than 40 patients described to date, of whom only a minority showed parkinsonism. All these cases presenting with SANDO-P were associated with mutations in the nuclear *POLG* gene, encoding the polymerase gamma (the only mtDNA polymerase in humans and animals). *POLG* defects are usually inherited recessively (as in our case) and lead, in turn, to mtDNA depletion in skeletal muscle and peripheral nerve tissue. The phenotype can vary widely, even within the same family, and can also encompass myopathy, seizures, and hearing loss, but the common clinical features appear to be sensory ataxia. Indeed, extraocular ophthalmoparesis cannot be the main feature in these patients, and only develop later in the course of the disease and often in mild forms. Other variable features include migraine and depression. The pathogenesis of parkinsonism occurring in this context is unknown, but obviously mitochondrial dysfunction is one possibility, since this is one of the mechanisms that is supposed to occur also in PD.

Suggested Readings

Hanisch F, Kornhuber M, Alston CL, Taylor RW, Deschauer M, Zierz S. SANDO syndrome in a cohort of 107 patients with CPEO and mitochondrial DNA deletions. *J Neurol Neurosurg Psychiatry*. 2015;86:630–4.

Milone M, Massie R. Polymerase gamma 1 mutations: clinical correlations. *Neurologist*. 2010;16:84–91.

 Video 64.1

There is an almost complete ophthalmoplegia on both horizontal and vertical plane. Gait is short-stepped and an episode of freezing occurs.

Ataxia Telangiectasia without Ataxia

Roberto Erro, Maria Stamelou, and Kailash P. Bhatia

Clinical History

This 18-year-old woman of Indian ancestry with no family history had a normal pregnancy, birth, and early milestones. She walked at 11 months and although a clumsy gait was noted during her childhood, she could compete with her peers at sports without any difficulties. She dated her first symptoms at the age of 15, when she noted an involuntary head turn to the right. Moreover, she developed speech difficulties and orofacial dyskinesias with involuntary movements of her jaw. She did not have any further complaints, namely she was not aware of any balance issues.

Examination

On examination (Video 65.1), it was found that eye movements were unremarkable, with both pursuits and saccades normal. She had generalized dystonia with predominant craniocervical distribution. In fact, there was torticollis to the right, jaw-opening dystonia, and dystonic tongue protrusion. Otherwise, her neurological examination was completely normal. In particular, there were no signs of cerebellar problems, with a normal gait including tandem gait.

Thorough physical examination revealed everything to be normal apart from a telangiectasia, which was visible on the left posterior pharyngeal wall.

General Remarks

As extensively discussed in Section 2 (cf. Case 25), a pronounced oromandibular dystonia would be unlikely for primary (or isolated) dystonia and is instead a red flag for secondary (i.e. tardive or post-anoxic) or heredodegenerative etiologies. Although the diagnostic work-up in cases like this one has been already described, here is an additional clinical feature (i.e. a leash of telangiectasia on the pharyngeal wall), which is of utmost importance to lead to the correct diagnosis.

Investigations and Diagnosis

Standard blood investigations revealed elevation of serum alpha-fetoprotein (406 IU/ml, normal≤30 IU/ml), while other tests including CEA, serum copper, ceruloplasmin, blood film for acanthocytes, white cell enzymes, uric acid, plasma amino acids, and urinary organic acids were normal. Brain MRI revealed mild cerebellar atrophy. Given the presence of telangiectasia suggesting an atypical presentation of AT, we further pursued genetic analysis of the *ATM* gene and an ATM Kinase assay. She was hence found homozygous for the missense mutation 590G>A in the *ATM* gene and functional studies showed that ATM level was reduced, the protein retained some kinase activity in vivo, as shown by the ability of the mutant ATM to autophosphorylate as well as phosphorylate downstream targets.

Special Remarks

AT is a rare autosomal recessive disorder caused by mutations in the *ATM* gene, which encodes a protein involved in the cellular DNA damage response and cell cycle checkpoint control. More than 400 mutations of the *ATM* have already been identified, most of which are private to single families. Owing to the large size of the gene, the utility of direct mutation screening as a diagnostic tool is limited and, in fact, genetic screening remains unsuccessful in up to 15 per cent of patients. Conversely, in vitro radiosensitivity assay of the ATM protein has a higher practical utility.

Classically, AT is characterized by progressive cerebellar ataxia beginning between 1 and 4 years of age, oculomotor apraxia or other ocular movement abnormalities, along with frequent infections (mainly pulmonary), immunodeficiency, an increased risk for malignancy (especially for leukemia and lymphoma), and obviously telangiectasia (a typical presentation of AT is shown in Video 65.2). Telangiectasias usually appear several years after the neurological onset and have been estimated to occur in up to 97 per cent of patients. These are usually found in the bulbar conjunctiva, but ear helices, the bridge of the nose, the butterfly area of the face, the back of the hands, axillae, popliteal and antecubital fossae should also be checked for the presence of dilated vessels.

AT is progressive, and affected individuals generally require a wheelchair by the age of 10 years, but there can be remarkable clinical heterogeneity, which arguably reflects the retained ATM activity. In very young children as well as in older individuals the neurological phenotype is often incomplete, and might include choreoathetosis and dystonia, thus rendering the differential diagnosis difficult. When the onset is in adulthood (sometimes referred to as variant-ATM), the phenotype is in fact dominated by movement disorders, including more commonly dystonia and myoclonus of the sub-cortical type and less frequently chorea or tremor, and ataxia is rarely the main compliant, despite being often the first sign to develop. The diagnostic challenge might also be due to the fact that MRI can show a normal-sized cerebellum for several years after the onset of ataxia. Hence, supportive laboratory features can be important and include elevated serum AFP, low T cell levels, and low serum levels of IgA, IgE, and IgG2. In some cases, like this one, cerebellar features can be completely absent. No treatment exists for AT and, given the central role of ATM in mobilizing the cellular response to DNA double-stranded breaks, there is a remarkable cancer susceptibility and sensitivity to ionizing radiation, which explains the approximately one-third of affected individuals who develop a cancer during their lifetimes. Patients who do not die from early incurable cancers or superimposed infections occasionally survive into their forties or fifties.

Suggested Readings

Charlesworth G, Mohire MD, Schneider SA, Stamelou M, Wood NW, Bhatia KP. Ataxia telangiectasia presenting as dopa-responsive cervical dystonia. *Neurology*. 2013;81:1148–51.

Chun HH, Gatti RA. Ataxia-telangiectasia, an evolving phenotype. *DNA Repair (Amst)*. 2004;3:1187–96.

Méneret A, Ahmar-Beaugendre Y, Rieunier G, et al. The pleiotropic movement disorders phenotype of adult ataxia-telangiectasia. *Neurology*. 2014;83:1087–95.

Video 65.1

There is dystonia, most prominent in her cervical region, with a sensory trick. Mild posturing and dystonic movements are seen in her upper limbs. There is no evidence of limb or gait ataxia. On the posterior pharyngeal wall a telangiectasia can be seen.

Video 65.2

Smooth pursuits are broken and there is gaze-evoked nystagmus as well as leashes of telangiectasia in the bulbar conjunctiva in both eyes. There is also mild ataxia and dysdiadochokinesia in the upper limbs.

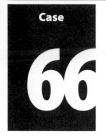

Case

66

Anti-Yo-Related Ataxia Misdiagnosed as MSA

George Dervenoulas, Leonidas Stefanis, and Maria Stamelou

Clinical History

This 76-year-old woman with no family history for any neurological disorders started noticing balance problems at the age of 73 years. She also complained of speech articulation problems. Her symptoms were progressive and about 2 years later she could walk only with the help of two caregivers, and her speech was almost unintelligible; she developed dysphagia and also a tremor in both arms (right>left) and head. At this stage, it was obvious that clinically she had a progressive cerebellar syndrome. Autonomic function tests showed a mild orthostatic hypotension and a mild urinary urgency. Magnetic resonance imaging showed mild cerebellar atrophy. On the basis of the age and a progressive cerebellar syndrome with autonomic dysfunction, the diagnosis of possible MSA-C was made, and the patient was prescribed levodopa with no benefit. She continued to worsen, particularly regarding her gait, speech, dysphagia, and severity of her tremor. Cognition was generally unaffected. Her medical history revealed that she was operated for adenocarcinoma of the left ovary in 2007 with total hysterectomy, colectomy, and chemotherapy. Since then she has been followed up regularly by her oncologist, and her tests were reported normal.

Examination

On examination (see Video 66.1), it was found that she had gaze-evoked nystagmus to the right>left and down-beat nystagmus. She had slightly slow saccades, cerebellar dysarthria, and occasionally a titubatory head tremor. She had limb ataxia more pronounced on the right, as well as a cerebellar tremor more on the right with slow frequency and high amplitude. She was unable to walk due to severe trunk and gait ataxia. There was no clear bradykinesia. She also had pyramidal signs, namely brisk reflexes in the lower limbs with bilateral extensor plantar responses.

General Remarks

Although a progressive cerebellar syndrome with pyramidal signs and autonomic involvement starting at an advanced age, with negative family history, would more likely support the diagnosis of a neurodegenerative disorder such as MSA-C or a SCA, there were some clues in this case that were unusual for that. The rapid progression leading to a wheelchair-bound state due to cerebellar ataxia in 2 years, the lack of parkinsonism, as well as the history of ovarian cancer, should prompt the exclusion of an immune-mediated cause, in particular paraneoplastic cerebellar degeneration. This is crucial, as these disorders may present before the appearance of a tumor and thus are important for treatment and prognosis, in contrast to neurodegenerative disorders, such as MSA or SCAs for which no effective treatment is available. Apart from the rapid progression, phenomenology was also a clue in this case. The severe cerebellar tremor involving also the head is rarely, if ever seen, in MSA. In contrast, the characteristic tremor in MSA is the poly-mini-myoclonus or a generally jerky tremor rather than a typical cerebellar, titubatory tremor.

Investigations and Diagnosis

As mentioned, a brain MRI scan showed moderate cerebellar atrophy (Figure 66.1). A DaT-Scan was normal, which made the diagnosis of MSA unlikely. Screening for paraneoplastic antibodies showed positive anti-Yo antibodies. A further screening for cancer was negative, and PET CT was negative. The diagnosis was revised to paraneoplastic cerebellar degeneration. The patient did not respond to immunotherapy and died around 10 months after diagnosis.

Special Remarks

Anti-Yo antibodies are one of the most common paraneoplastic antibodies. Clinically, most patients present with a subacute and mostly severe pancerebellar

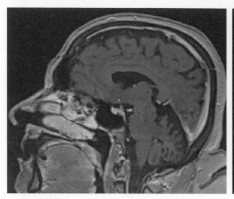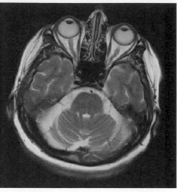

Figure 66.1 Sagittal (left panel) and axial (right panel) slices showing mild cerebellar atrophy.

syndrome with truncal and appendicular ataxia, dysarthria, and nystagmus; other signs and symptoms may include pyramidal signs, peripheral neuropathy, dysphagia, diplopia, and cognitive impairment. Median age at onset is 61 years (range, 26–85) and almost all patients are female. In the majority of patients, the onset of symptoms precede the tumour diagnosis by months or even years. Accordingly, regular screening for malignant tumours is required; however, in some cases, neoplasms remain occult and can be detected only on autopsy.

MRI often shows cerebellar atrophy after some weeks or months but may be normal at disease onset. CSF often shows lymphocytic pleocytosis, oligoclonal bands, an increased CSF/serum ratio and elevated total protein levels.

Anti-Yo antibodies are usually associated with malignant gynaecological tumours (ovary, breast, mesovarium, fallopian tube, uterus, or cervix), which are often confined to the involved organs or local lymph nodes. Rarely, other tumours have been found, including lung cancer. In the few male anti-Yo-positive patients, this was associated with adenocarcinomas (prostate, esophagus, stomach, or intestine).

Treatment of the underlying tumour is the mainstay of disease management. Immunosuppression has mostly no or only minor effect, and has been reported beneficial only in some cases, especially if treatment was initiated shortly after disease onset. The median survival time in anti-Yo-positive patients is 22 months, but longer survival (up to 164 months) has been reported. Prognosis is also determined by the type of the underlying tumour; however, in 40 per cent of the cases, the cerebellar degeneration is the cause of death.

Suggested Readings

Höftberger R, Rosenfeld MR, Dalmau J. Update on neurological paraneoplastic syndromes. *Curr Opin Oncol.* 2015;27:489–95.

Mitoma H, Hadjivassiliou M, Honnorat J. Guidelines for treatment of immune-mediated cerebellar ataxias. *Cerebellum Ataxias.* 2015;2:14.

 Video 66.1

There is limb ataxia, more pronounced on the right, as well as a cerebellar tremor more on the right with slow frequency and high amplitude.

Late Onset Spinocerebellar Ataxia: SCA3

67

Christos Ganos

Clinical History

This 59-year-old woman of German descent presented with an 11-year-long history of progressive balance difficulties. At symptom onset, she had found it difficult to walk a straight line. Over the ensuing period, and as symptoms progressed, others had commented that her gait had become unusual and unsteady, as if she were 'under the influence of alcohol'. She developed difficulties writing, as well as speech problems. At the age of 55, she had further experienced stiffness in her legs, associated with painful cramps and paraesthesias, particularly when lying down. During the same period, she developed increased urinary urgency leading to incontinence. She also manifested symptoms of orthostatic hypotension and she has, therefore, been treated with midodrine hydrochloride (2.5 mg bd). At the age of 57, she required a walking aid to maintain her balance. There was a positive family history; the patient's father had developed similar symptoms and had become wheelchair-bound by the age of 50.

Examination

There was broken smooth pursuit with gaze-evoked nystagmus. Saccadic latency and speed were normal for voluntary and reflexive saccades. However, there was clear saccadic dysmetria, with both hypo- and hypermetria when presented a visual target. Vestibulo-occular reflex and its suppression were impaired. There were occasional periorbicular fasciculations during examination. There was clear cerebellar dysarthria. There was clear leg spasticity with prominent hip adductor activation. Plantars were extensor bilaterally. Vibration perception over the medial malleolus was reduced bilaterally. There was no bradykinesia. There was clear truncal ataxia, as well as upper limb ataxia with intention tremor and dysmetria. Gait was unsteady, with a mixture of ataxia and spasticity (segments of the examination are demonstrated in Video 67.1A).

General Remarks

This lady developed a slowly progressive (spino)cerebellar disorder at the age of 48. The first differential diagnostic consideration to make from the patient's history is related to the temporal dynamic of symptom progression, which was ongoing and over a period of 11 years, i.e. chronic. This renders acute or subacute causes of spinocerebellar syndromes, such as vascular, infectious (e.g. abscess), or autoimmune (e.g. post-infectious, paraneoplastic) unlikely. The second consideration relates to the presence of family history for cerebellar disorders (patient's father was affected). This allows distinguishing between sporadic and hereditary ataxias, shifting, in this particular case, the diagnostic probability towards the latter category. Within the spectrum of hereditary ataxias, age of onset (early usually considered <25 years vs. adult or late onset) should be considered next. Typically, early onset hereditary ataxias are of autosomal-recessive inheritance, whereas familial ataxias with adult/late onset are usually inherited in an autosomal-dominant manner. The patient's age of symptom onset and the affected father corroborate this diagnostic rule. This notwithstanding, exceptions may occur (e.g. late and very late onset Friedreich's ataxia). Further, mitochondrial disorders, which usually also affect the cerebellum, may present with a large variety of symptoms at any age, but in most cases some of the signs usually manifest from a young age. For the presented case, it appears that a late onset, autosomal-dominant inherited SCA would be the most likely scenario.

SCAs comprise an expanding spectrum of different genetic disorders with the phenotypic overlap of progressive spinocerebellar degeneration. Although particular syndromic associations cluster around certain SCAs more frequent than others (e.g. retinal degeneration in SCA7, prominent cognitive symptoms in SCA17, myoclonus in SCA14) most characteristics do overlap for most SCAs. Noteworthy, some of the most common SCAs (e.g. SCA1, 2, 3) but also SCA6, 7, 17, and DRPLA are due to pathological repeat expansions (polyQ-SCAs), whereas other, rarer SCAs are due to point mutations, rearrangements, or non-coding repeat expansions. Importantly, patients with PolyQ-SCAs require earlier walking assistance and have shorter disease duration than patients from the other categories. The presented patient required a walking aid within the first 10 years of her illness. This hints towards a polyQ-SCA. SCA3 is the most common SCA worldwide, with some minor exceptions depending on the exact geographic location of origin (e.g. SCA2 in Cuba).

Investigations and Diagnosis

Routine laboratory blood work, including Vitamin E levels, was unremarkable. CSF examination was equally unrevealing. Eye examination was normal. Nerve conduction studies showed evidence of sensory neuropathy in the legs. Repeated brain MRI had indicated the presence of infratentorial, most prominent cerebellar, atrophy.

Given the aforementioned differential diagnostic approach, common polyQ-SCAs were tested (SCA1,2,3). A pathological repeat expansion for the SCA3 (ataxin-3) gene in one allele was found (69/23 repeats) and the diagnosis of SCA3 was made. Noteworthy, due to the increased hip adductor spasticity, symptomatic treatment with botulinum toxin injections in the long adductor muscle bilaterally was commenced. This led to a drastic reduction of spasticity-associated leg pain and increase in functional range of motion (Video 67.1B). As expected, there was no effect of botulinum toxin injection treatment on gait ataxia.

Special Remarks

SCA3 (also termed Machado-Joseph disease after two of the three original families described) is the most common of all SCAs. Affected individuals have pathological CAG trinucleotide repeat expansions in ataxin-3 gene (> 52; shorter pathological expansions recently reported). As also in other polyQ-SCAs, there is an inverse correlation between age at symptom onset and length of expanded repeats. Although spinocerebellar degeneration is the hallmark feature of SCA3, depending on manifesting age, different clinical subphenotypes have been described. Accordingly, the first subphenotype with a younger age of onset (10–30 years) has a rather rapid progression, prominent extrapyramidal features, particularly dystonia, as well as pyramidal abnormalities, whereas the degree of cerebellar dysfunction may vary. Subphenotype II is described to have a later onset (20–50 years) and is characterized by a classic spinocerebellar syndrome (i.e. ataxia and spasticity), as in the presented case. Subphenotype III (onset > 40 years) has a relative slow progression and presents with a combination of cerebellar symptoms and polyneuropathy. Beyond these subphenotypes, other presentations include a pure cerebellar syndrome, a (levodopa responsive) parkinsonian (+ ataxia) phenotype, as well as spastic paraparesis being the predominant symptom. Dysautonomia, restless legs syndrome, dysphagia, and urinary incontinence are frequent findings in nearly all patients in the course of the disorder. Unsurprisingly, neuropathological changes in SCA3 patients extend well beyond the cerebellum to affect cortical and subcortical areas, including the basal ganglia. To date, treatment remains symptomatic.

Suggested Readings

Durr A. Autosomal dominant cerebellar ataxias: polyglutamine expansions and beyond. *Lancet Neurol.* 2010;9:885–94.

Jacobi H, Bauer P, Giunti P, et al. The natural history of spinocerebellar ataxia type 1, 2, 3, and 6: a 2-year follow-up study. *Neurology.* 2011;77:1035–41.

Nakano KK, Dawson DM, Spence A. Machado disease: a hereditary ataxia in Portuguese immigrants to Massachusetts. *Neurology.* 1972;22:49–55.

Video 67.1

A: This patient has truncal ataxia as well as upper limb dysmetria (left>right) and dysdiadochokinesis. There is leg spasticity with prominent involvement of the hip adductors. Spastic-ataxic gait with prominent truncal ataxia is shown. B: The same patient 6 months later after having been treated with botulinum toxin injections into both long adductor muscles.

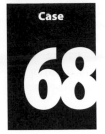

Ataxia with Splenomegaly: Niemann-Pick Disease Type C

Roberto Erro and Kailash P. Bhatia

Clinical History

This 47-year-old man with no family history was referred for an 8-year history of incoordination on the left side of his body, which he first noted when playing football. He was also complaining of an occasional tremor as well as an altered sensation in his left hand with a sense of pins and needles in the palm. Moreover, his hearing and vision were deteriorating. His wife mentioned that he has become forgetful, more short tempered and had not been socializing. There were also problems in concentrating, but he was still working and supporting his family. Over the last year he further developed two episodes of lethargy, vomiting, and epistaxis.

Examination

On examination, it was found that he had difficulty initiating saccades, which were also slow. On the vertical plane, his eyes would not move vertically up but rather in a circuitous route, reminiscent of the 'round-the-house' sign. Smooth pursuits were normal. There was excessive blinking. There was mild dysdiadochokinesia with his left hand. On finger–nose tapping he showed some clumsiness with his left hand, but there was no dysmetria. He had slowness when performing repetitive movements, but no true decrement could be observed on finger tapping. Reflexes were brisk and symmetrical. There was some minor subjective reduction in pin-prick on the median aspect of the left hand, but otherwise sensory testing was normal. Gait was slow and he had some difficulties in tandem walking. The remaining neurological examination was normal, but on physical examination he was found to have splenomegaly.

General Remarks

Despite the paucity of neurological signs on examination, the presence of splenomegaly – along with the history of lethargy, vomiting, and epistaxis – is of utmost importance. This in fact suggests a disorder where a neurological involvement occurs in the context of a systemic disease. The combination of cerebellar symptoms with splenomegaly should promptly raise the suspicion of NPC. In line with this there was also the evidence of the 'round-the-house' sign on ocular examination. Other rare late onset lysosomal storage diseases can produce splenomegaly and a neurological involvement, the diagnosis of which depends on the presence of specific enzymatic deficiency in peripheral blood leukocytes or cultured fibroblasts. Alternatively, it is important to remember that severe hepatic failure can in turn lead to splenomegaly and, in this context, WD should be excluded. However, this would be unlikely since this type of eye movement abnormalities are usually not seen in WD.

Investigations and Diagnosis

Given the high suspicion of a lysosomal storage disorder, a bone marrow biopsy was performed which showed foamy cells in keeping with a diagnosis of NPC, which was then confirmed with the filipin test that proved excessive storage of free cholesterol. A brain MRI was performed which turned out to be normal.

Special Remarks

NPC is a rare, progressive genetic lysosomal lipid storage disease caused by mutations in either the *NPC1* (up to 95 per cent of cases) or *NPC2* (approximately 5 per cent of cases) gene. It is a highly heterogeneous disease, with variable age at onset and characterized by visceral, neurological, and psychiatric manifestations that can present alone or in combination. Symptoms at onset might be subtle and non-specific, and in fact there is an average delay in diagnosis of 5–6 years from onset of neurological symptoms. Yet, there are combinations of symptoms that are strongly suggestive of NPC, and these include splenomegaly and vertical supranuclear gaze palsy, ataxia, or schizophrenia-like psychosis. On the other hand, as stated earlier, not all patients develop organomegaly and therefore NPC should be considered also in early adults presenting with ataxia or dystonia and eye movement abnormalities, particularly vertical supranuclear gaze palsy. The disease can be very heterogeneous and additional neurological symptoms can occur, including seizures, gelastic cataplexy, hearing loss, and cognitive decline. Progressive cognitive decline, which always occurs in patients with NPC as the disease progresses, usually manifests as memory and executive impairment in adult patients. Disease prognosis mainly correlates with the age at onset of the neurological signs, with early onset forms progressing faster.

NPC diagnosis is confirmed on biochemical (filipin staining) and genetic testing for those patients where fibroblast culture has yielded equivocal results. The diagnosis should be promptly made in order to start the treatment with Miglustat. It is the only disease-specific approved therapy for the treatment of progressive neurological manifestations of NPC. Miglustat has been shown to improve or stabilize key parameters of neurological disease progression both in children and adult patients and should be initiated at the earliest signs of neurological manifestations.

Suggested Readings

Mengel E, Klünemann HH, Lourenço CM, et al. Niemann-Pick disease type C symptomatology: an expert-based clinical description. *Orphanet J Rare Dis*. 2013;8:166.

Patterson MC, Hendriksz CJ, Walterfang M, Sedel F, Vanier MT, Wijburg F. Recommendations for the diagnosis and management of Niemann-Pick disease type C: an update. *Mol Genet Metab*. 2012;106:330–44.

Sévin M, Lesca G, Baumann N, et al. The adult form of Niemann-Pick disease type C. *Brain*. 2007;130:120–33.

Index